The Powered Wheelchair Training Guide

The Powered Wheelchair Training Guide

**Written by Peter Axelson, Jean Minkel,
Anita Perr and Denise Yamada**

Illustrations by Clay Butler

PAX Press
Minden, NV

This training guide was completed with a grant from the Paralyzed Veterans of America's Spinal Cord Injury Education and Training Foundation.

The illustrations were completed with funding from Beneficial Designs, Inc.

Designed by Kathleen Wong, Peter Axelson, Wayne Wright, and Jeff Conger

PAX Press is a division of Beneficial Designs, Inc.
P.O. Box 69
Minden, Nevada 89423-0069

ISBN 1-882632-11-7

Copyright © 2002 by PAX Press. All rights reserved. No part of this work covered by the copyright hereon may be reproduced or used in any form or by any means – graphic, electronic, or mechanical, including photocopying, recording, taping, or information storage and retrieval systems – without prior written consent of the publisher.

Printed in the United States of America

Table of Contents

Acknowledgments	ix
Introduction	x
How to Use this Book	x
Warnings	xi

Chapter 1: Getting to Know Your Wheels — 1

1.1 The Owner's Manual — 2

1.2 Determining the Powered Wheelchair Type Best for You — 3
- Wheelchair Types — 3
- Drive Configurations — 5

1.3 Specifying the Seating Components and Control Input Device — 7
- Selecting and Ordering Your Powered Wheelchair — 7
- Seating Dimensions and Components — 7
- Joystick Type — 11
- Alternate Controls — 12

1.4 Seating Setup and Wheel Adjustments — 13
- Seat Surface Angle Adjustment — 13
- Back Angle Adjustment — 14
- Drive Wheel Position Adjustment — 14
- Arm Support Height Adjustment — 15
- Caster Adjustments — 15
- Foot Support Adjustment — 16
- Seat Height Adjustment — 16

1.5 Joystick Setup, Adjustments and Operation — 17
- Joystick Positioning — 17
- Joystick Handles — 17
- Dealer Programmable Drive Performance Adjustments — 18
- Reversal of Controls — 20
- User Adjustable Settings and Joystick Operations — 20
- Checking Your Stability with a Spotter — 22

Chapter 2: General Skills — 25

2.1 Asking for Help — 26
- Defining "Assistance" — 26
- Who Can Help? — 26
- How to Ask for Help — 28
- Manually Rolling Your Wheelchair — 29
- Describing Safe Body Mechanics to the Spotter or Assistant — 29
- When You Do Not Want or Need Assistance — 29
- Experiencing New Environments — 29

2.2 Learning Your Limits — 30
- Techniques for Keeping Your Weight Back — 30
- Techniques for Keeping Your Weight Forward — 32
- When You are Learning Your Limits — 33

Table of Contents

2.3 Relieving Pressure — 34
- Forward Weight Shift — 34
- Side-to-Side Weight Shift — 35
- Push Up Weight Shift — 36
- Weight Shift Through Powered Seating — 36

2.4 Reaching, Bending and Lifting — 38
- Reaching Sideways — 38
- Reaching Forward — 39

2.5 Main Wheel and Caster Management — 41
- Wheel Position — 41
- Wheel Size — 42
- Composition — 42
- Condition — 42
- Caster Management and Caster Trail — 43
- Type of Caster — 44
- Caster Flutter — 44

Chapter 3: Navigation Skills — 45

3.1 Smooth Surfaces — 47
- Crossing Smooth Surfaces — 47

3.2 Thresholds and Obstacles — 48
- Foot Support Clearance — 48
- Crossing a Door Threshold or Obstacle — 49

3.3 Doorways and Tight Environments — 53
- Manual Swinging Doors — 54
- Manual Sliding Doors — 56
- Doors in a Sequence — 57
- Double-leaf Doors — 57
- Narrow Doors — 58
- Automatic Doors — 58
- Revolving Doors and Turnstiles — 59
- Doors with Objects Around Them — 59
- Tight Environments — 59
- Vans — 62

3.4 Rough Terrain — 63
- Hard, Uneven Surfaces — 63
- Soft Surfaces — 64

3.5 Ramps — 66
- Going Up a Ramp — 66
- Going Down a Ramp — 67
- Very Steep Ramps — 69
- Telescoping or Portable Ramps — 69
- Turning Around on a Ramp — 69
- Grade Transitions — 70

3.6 Cross Slopes — 71
- Walkways and Hills with Cross Slopes — 71
- Curb Ramps — 72
- Driveway Crossings — 73

3.7 Curbs and Steps — 74
- Going Up Curbs or Steps — 74
- Going Down Curbs — 77

3.8 Elevators and Platform Lifts — 80
- Catching an Elevator — 80
- Entering and Exiting an Elevator — 82
- Platform Lifts — 84

3.9	**Tracks and Grates**	**85**
	Crossing Railroad and Trolley Tracks	85
	Crossing Grates	86

Chapter 4: Emergency Skills — 89

4.1	**Stairs**	**90**
	Going Up Stairs	91
	Going Down Stairs	91
4.2	**Falling and Getting Up**	**93**
	Falling	93
	Battery Acid	94
	Getting Up	94
4.3	**Electromagnetic Compatibility**	**97**
	Sources of Electromagnetic Energy	98
	Dealing with EMI	98
4.4	**Evacuation Procedures**	**100**
	Creating an Emergency Plan	101
	Personal Emergency	101

Chapter 5: Special Circumstances — 103

5.1	**Planning Your Route**	**104**
	Transit Stops	104
	Trains and Automobiles	105
	Airplanes	105
	Rental Vehicles	105
5.2	**Crossing Streets**	**106**
	Understand the Local Driver Mentality	106
	Examining Street Terrain	106
	Crossing at a Crosswalk	107
	Crossing at Mid-block	108
5.3	**Nighttime Safety**	**110**
	General Pointers	110
	Emergency Equipment	111
	Protect Yourself	112
	Moving Around	112
5.4	**Hiking**	**113**
	Hiking Hazards	113
	Prepare for Your Trip	113
	Take Precautions	114
	Asking for Assistance	114
5.5	**Traveling**	**116**
	Travel Planning Tips	116
	Hotel Rooms	117
	Restrooms	117
	New Environments	118
	Other Hazards	118
5.6	**Weather**	**119**
	Precipitation	119
	Sun	121
	Wind	121

Table of Contents

5.7 Transportation — 122
- General Considerations and Safety Issues — 122
- Transferring In and Out of Your Wheelchair — 123
- Riding in Vehicles While in Your Wheelchair — 124
- Air Travel — 126

Chapter 6: Body Mechanics — 129

6.1 Protecting Yourself — 130
- Body Position — 130
- Using Safe Body Mechanics — 131

6.2 Setting Limits and Offering Help — 134
- How to Say "No" — 134
- Offering Assistance — 134

Appendix A: The Americans with Disabilities Act of 1990 — 137

Appendix B: Specialty Powered Wheelchairs and Accessories — 139

Appendix C: References and Resources — 148

Acknowledgments

The writing of this book was completed with a grant from the Paralyzed Veterans of America's Spinal Cord Injury Education and Training Foundation. The illustrations for this book were funded by Beneficial Designs, Inc.

I wish to thank the focus group participants and manuscript reviewers whose assistance and expertise made it possible to develop this training guide.

Foster Anderson	Shared Adventures
Brian Arakaki	St. Jude Medical Center
Marty Ball	Ti Sport
Dev Banerjee	Penny and Giles Drives Technology
Gina Bertocci	University of Pittsburgh
Frankie Cassaday	Craig Hospital
Rory Cooper	Highland Drive VA Medical Center, Pittsburgh
Jim Ernst	Burke Inc. / Leisure-Lift
Tom Finch	TEFTEC Corporation
John Fulland	SINTEF Unimed
Gail Gilinsky	Craig Hospital
Gil Haury	Invacare Corporation
Michael Heckrotte	Precision Calibration, Inc.
Susan Johnson-Taylor	Rehabilitation Institute of Chicago
Kay Koch-Hurst	Texas Scottish Rite Hospital for Children
Betti Krapfl	Craig Hospital
David Kreutz	Shepherd Spinal Center
Lupo Quitoriano	Paralyzed Veterans of America, University of Southern Mississippi
Dennis Rollinger	Radiometrics Midwest
Larry Schneider	University of Michigan Transportation Research Institute
Julie Steward	University of Kansas
Chris Wenner	Powered wheelchair user

I wish to also thank Dr. David Gray and the students in his Assistive Technology course in the Program in Occupational Therapy at the Washington University School of Medicine who reviewed the manuscript: Linda Bernal, Rashida Byams, Hillery Cleveland, Jessica Davinroy, Sarah Ebelhar, Kathleen Gwost, Jennifer Haga, Kimberly Hannon, Elizabeth Hawkins-Chernof, Benjamin Haynes, Rachel Heiligman, Jennifer Herron, Heather Lavenburg, Kerri Morgan, Theresa Polefko, Darci Redmond, Amanda Scroggins, Tasha Smith, Sara Stock, Emily Stork, Jennifer Struna, and Deanna Venvertloh.

This book could not have been completed without the hard work and endless hours of editing by Beneficial Designs staff: Mindy Pasternak, Kathleen Wong, Stacy Rose, Jenny Tuohy and Schelly Jackson.

Thanks also to Ray Buetens of Slub Design for his Quark expertise and assistance with the book layout.

Clay Butler deserves special recognition for his illustration work that brings imagination, life and humor to this serious topic.

I want to thank my coauthors, Jean and Anita, with their many, many years of experience teaching this stuff to users, therapists and caregivers, for reviewing the content again and again.

And finally to Denise for her attention to so many details and her incredible organizational skills. The project would never have been completed without her support.

I hope you enjoy this guide, that it brings you the information you need, that it helps you build confidence in your wheelchair driving abilities, and most important of all, that it teaches you safe and independent mobility.

Peter Axelson

Introduction

Those who use wheelchairs for mobility and transportation depend heavily on their wheelchair maneuvering skills to complete basic living tasks. The many kinds of environments people encounter daily present complex skill and safety challenges to wheelchair riders and their helpers. Unfortunately, many people have not been properly trained in the safe and efficient use of their wheelchairs. Improper skills commonly result in falls and serious injury to wheelchair riders and their assistants.

This book was designed to be used by wheelchair users, their families, friends, caregivers and anyone else who might need comprehensive information about powered wheelchair skills. The illustrated instructions provide guidance for wheelchair users on how to negotiate indoor environments, obstacles, and outdoor terrain. General hints to prepare for traveling, emergencies, and other situations are also included. In addition, this training guide provides instructions on how to assist someone with a technique and describes the progressions for learning new maneuvers. The principles discussed will help readers learn good wheelchair riding and assisting habits, which are applicable to any mobility skills they might develop in the future.

The skills and information in this guide will hopefully help increase the independence of wheelchair users, decrease the number of wheelchair accidents caused by the lack of education and training, and limit the frustration caused by those receiving or giving inadequate or improper assistance. The wheelchair skills and instructions in this book were compiled with the assistance of wheelchair users and rehabilitation professionals. These experienced individuals provided input on the wheelchair techniques, text content, and illustrations.

How to Use this Book

We recommend that new wheelchair users or those who have limited familiarity with powered chairs read this guide thoroughly to learn about all aspects of their use. Those more experienced or familiar with wheelchairs may prefer to skim the table of contents to locate specific topics.

Many of the illustrations contain white and/or black arrows. The wider, white arrows indicate the direction of travel. The thin, black arrows indicate the direction the wheelchair rider should move the joystick.

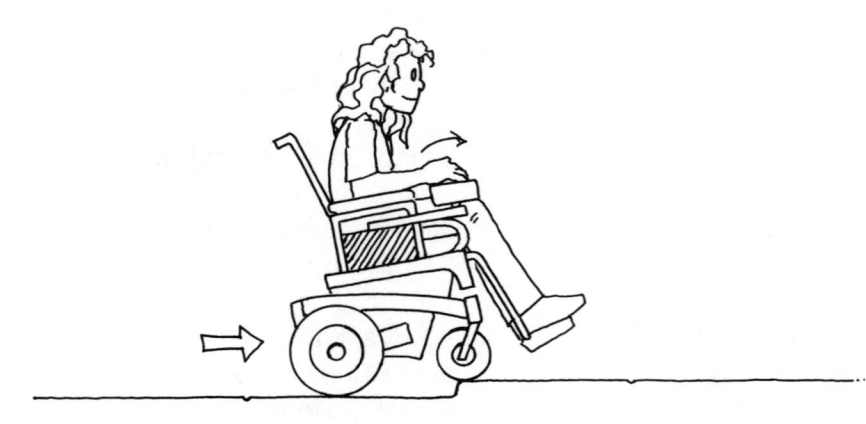

Warnings

Any opinions, conclusions or recommendations expressed herein include those of the focus group participants, wheelchair experts and manuscript reviewers consulted for the book and do not necessarily reflect the views or policies of the organizations that funded the development of this book. Beneficial Designs, Inc. and the Paralyzed Veterans of America do not endorse or recommend any of the specific skills described in this guide, and are not responsible for any injuries or deaths that may occur as a result of practicing or performing these techniques.

We attempted to incorporate all powered wheelchair skills that we are aware of into this book, regardless of the potential hazards associated with performing them. Many of the skills described in this book require a considerable amount of skill, balance and/or strength to perform safely. Many of the riskier techniques described, such as going up and down stairs, should only be used in emergencies. Performing these techniques incorrectly could result in severe injuries or death if you do not have the requisite assistance. For some people, just falling from a wheelchair could result in severe injury or death.

If you attempt these maneuvers, enlist the help of a physical or occupational therapist or RESNA certified assistive technology supplier (ATS) or practitioner (ATP) who is experienced in wheelchair training. Use extreme caution while practicing and performing the techniques described in this book. Always enlist physically capable spotters when attempting more difficult techniques or performing skills for the first time.

Be aware that assisting a wheelchair user as a spotter or assistant could result in severe injury to you. Obtain training from a physical or occupational therapist or a RESNA certified ATP to learn proper lifting and assisting skills.

CHAPTER 1

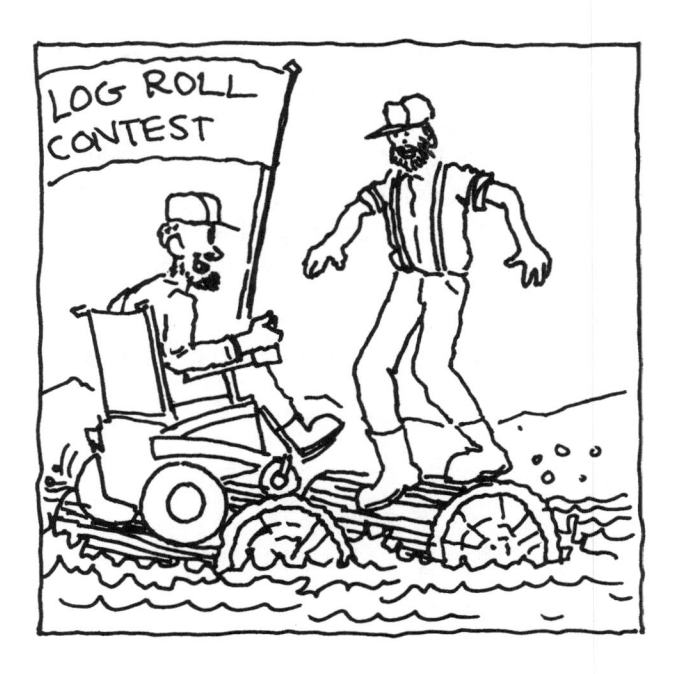

Getting to Know Your Wheels

In this Chapter

1.1	The Owner's Manual	2
1.2	Determining the Powered Wheelchair Type Best for You	3
1.3	Specifying the Seating Components and Control Input Device	7
1.4	Seating Setup and Wheel Adjustments	13
1.5	Joystick Setup, Adjustments and Operation	17

If you're a new wheelchair user, you'll want to get to know your new wheels. Chapter 1 provides basic information so you can begin using your wheelchair as effectively as possible.

Chapter One: Getting to Know Your Wheels

Section 1.1

The Owner's Manual

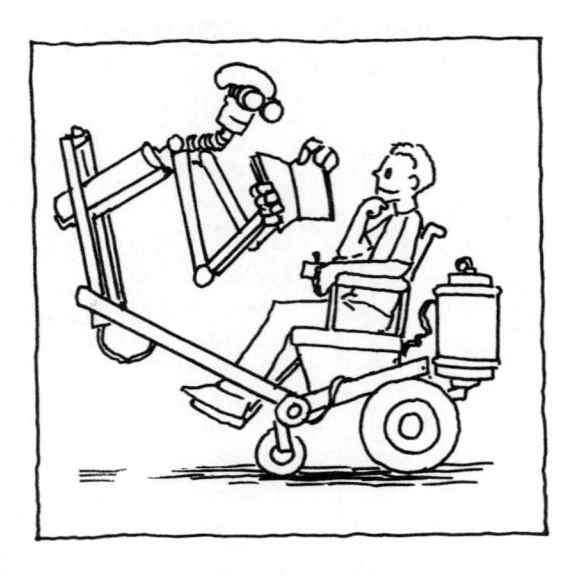

As with all new gadgets, you should read and familiarize yourself with the owner's manual before using your wheelchair. Although different wheelchair models may seem similar, each has a unique set of features and adjustments whose secrets lie inside the booklet that came with the chair. Take the time to understand your wheelchair before attempting to maneuver in complex environments. Keep in mind, you could be injured and/or your wheelchair damaged if your wheelchair is set up or operated improperly.

Read the manual from cover to cover. The information contained in wheelchair owner's manuals is very important. Most manuals include information about:

- Assembly instructions
- Adjustments your supplier should make
- Adjustments you can make
- General safety and handling characteristics
- Operating characteristics unique to your chair
- Wheelchair parts list
- Available accessories
- Maintenance procedures
- Warranty

If you have any questions, comments or concerns about the assembly, adjustment, wheelchair handling, or anything in the owner's manual, contact your wheelchair supplier or manufacturer. Do not attempt to adjust components if you do not fully understand the instructions in the manual, as your actions might create unsafe conditions or void the warranty. Do not use your wheelchair until it has been properly assembled and adjusted.

Read the owner's manual from cover to cover.

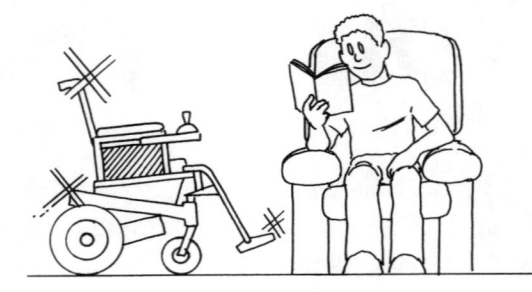

Section 1.2

Determining the Powered Wheelchair Type Best for You

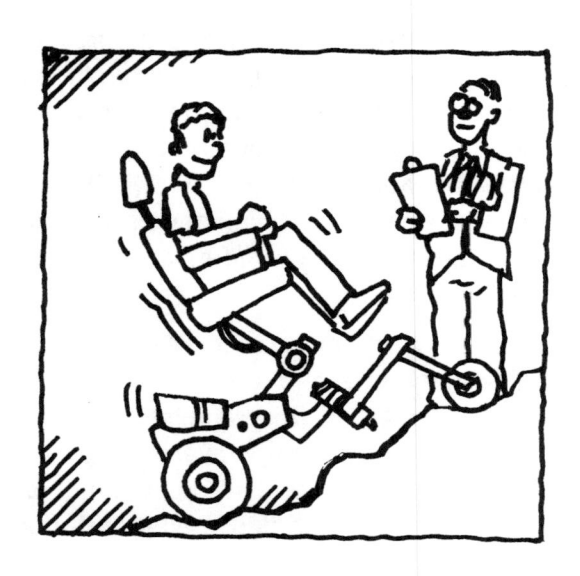

Wheelchair Types

As with the automobile, inventors have developed many different styles and models of wheelchairs. Each is designed for a different purpose, and permits different types of adjustments to be made.

Changes easily made on standard powered wheelchairs include:
- foot support positioning (typically only length adjustment)
- arm support adjustment
- joystick positioning
- upholstery replacement

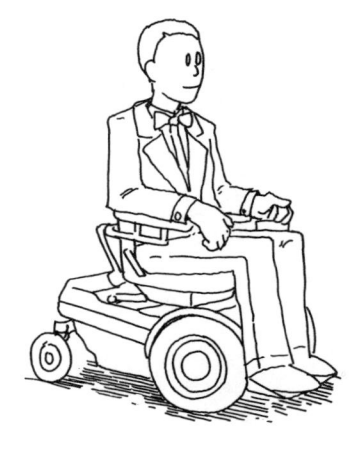

This is a front-wheel drive powered wheelchair with a power base.

There are many types of powered wheelchairs currently on the market. They generally fall into two main categories: scooters and powered wheelchairs.

Scooters

Scooters usually have three or four wheels and have a seat that is mounted on a pedestal attached to the floor of the scooter. One main difference between a scooter and a conventional powered wheelchair is the way it is steered. On a conventional powered wheelchair, an electronic control input device, such as a joystick, causes different amounts of power to go to each of the rear wheels to control both speed and direction. On a scooter, users generally hold handlebars at the end of a tiller that is attached to the front wheel (or wheels) to mechanically turn the wheelchair. Four-wheeled scooters typically have the front wheels connected together such that turning the tiller left and right causes the front wheels to turn left and right together. While turning the tiller often controls the direction of movement, the speed of the scooter is usually controlled with a lever attached to the handlebars, which is pressed with the thumbs or another part of the hand. Scooters often require more arm movement and hand function to operate than traditional powered wheelchairs. Scooters do not typically provide foot positioning to accommodate users that have no leg function. The seating on a scooter is typically not designed to accommodate someone with poor trunk stability. For these reasons, scooters are generally used by persons who have the ability to walk, but who may be limited on how far they can stand or walk.

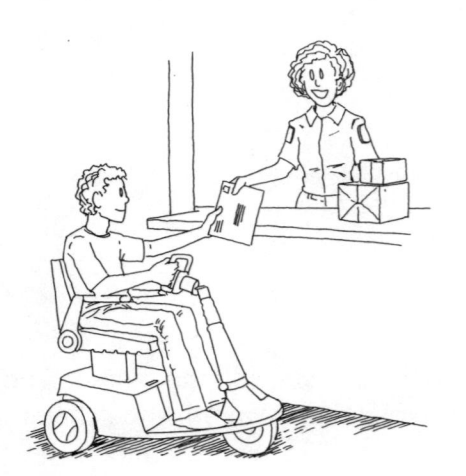

This is a three-wheeled scooter.

The seats of most scooters rotate and lock into position. The seat is often rotated and locked when the person is transferring onto and off the scooter. If the person cannot get close enough to a table or other object when approaching it from the front, the user can rotate the pivoting seat, to the side or all the way around to the rear. Some scooters also have elevating seats that may be adjusted, depending on the height of the user or the activity performed. Many manufacturers of cushions and back supports make products that can easily be placed on the seat of the scooter.

One of the positive features of scooters is that their overall wheelbase tends to be longer, providing greater stability in the fore-aft direction. That length however, can make it difficult to maneuver in some situations. A scooter may be more stable side-to-side than a powered wheelchair, depending on the width of the scooter. The manual linkage for the tiller steering allows the scooter user to turn rapidly and this can cause the scooter to begin to tip to the side. If not corrected immediately by turning the tiller back in the other direction, the scooter could tip over.

Powered wheelchairs with power bases

When talking about powered wheelchairs, people usually picture a powered wheelchair with a power base. They differ from scooters in their design and operation. Power base wheelchairs have a base that houses the motors, batteries and wheels, along with a seating system that is mounted on top of the base. Most powered wheelchair bases have at least four wheels. While scooters are steered using a tiller that is mechanically linked to the front wheel(s), power base wheelchairs can be controlled using a variety of input switches. The most common control input device is a joystick that is operated by the hand. Powered wheelchairs can also be controlled using joysticks operated by other parts of the body, or by a variety of single or multiple switches, including sip and puff breath-activated ones. Many people who are unable to operate scooters due to limited arm function, are able to use traditional powered wheelchairs.

Powered wheelchairs come in a variety of drive wheel types: front-wheel drive, mid-wheel drive and rear-wheel drive. There are also a variety of specialty powered wheelchairs. These fall into several categories, including stair climbing powered chair bases that are intended for independent or attendant operation, those that are able to move laterally, and those designed for off-road use.

Powered chairs for traveling

Due to the weight of most power base chairs, transportation is a major consideration. Users of power base chairs often prefer using a modified van or mini van for their personal vehicle. There are a limited number of powered chairs available that are ideal for travel. These chairs differ from the typical power base chairs that do not fold. They are easier to remove the batteries, have smaller drive wheels and can be quickly folded to put in the back of a vehicle.

Traveling powered chairs more closely resemble a folding manual wheelchair equipped with motors and batteries. The folding frame allows for easier transport. The batteries are often housed in separate boxes with easy to separate electrical connectors, which facilitate dismantling the chair. After removing the batteries and the battery tray, the chair can fold. The motors and controller are usually still mounted to the frame, which results in at least one heavy component to be lifted into and out of a vehicle. While dismantling and folding the chair would not likely be a daily activity, knowing a chair *can* be folded and transported in a car, may be very useful for some users.

In terms of durability, generally traveling powered chairs are not designed to be as durable as power base chairs. You will need to consider the trade-off of car transportation and your power mobility driving needs – light-duty versus heavy-duty use.

Add-on power systems and power-assist wheels

Two other options are available if you are considering power mobility. Both of these product types – add-on power systems and power-assist wheels – use a manual wheelchair frame as the base structure.

Add-on power systems are a means of converting a manual wheelchair frame into a power mobility device. Several methods are available, including a conversion unit that operates like a scooter with tiller steering, and another unit that uses specialized wheels, a battery pack and a joystick to create a more traditional powered chair conversion.

Wheelchairs with power-assist wheels can be considered as a transitional product between manual mobility and power mobility. Most wheelchairs with power-assist wheels are sold as complete wheelchairs. Power-assist wheels have motors inside of the wheels that amplify the push of the user on the handrim – the switch that tells the wheel to go forward. Depending on how hard the user pushes on the handrim, the wheel puts out more or less power to amplify the user's push. The power-assist wheels extend the length of the roll from a single push. The effect is to travel longer distances with less effort.

While either option may be suitable to meet a person's needs, these devices are not designed to be as durable or as powerful as a power base chair.

Drive Configurations

Front-, rear- and mid-wheel drive powered chairs

Front-wheel drive chairs have large drive wheels in the front of the chair with casters (usually smaller wheels) in the rear. Front-wheel drive chairs were first introduced in Europe and are now becoming more popular in the U.S., where rear-wheel drive chairs have traditionally been most predominant.

Rear-wheel drive chairs have the larger wheels in the rear with the casters in front.

In the mid 1990's, several manufacturers introduced **mid-wheel drive** powered chairs. These wheelchairs have the main drive wheel centered under the user's center of mass. Mid-wheel drive powered chairs have six wheels: two drive wheels, a pair of casters and a pair of anti-tipping wheels. The casters and anti-tippers may be mounted either in the front or the rear of the chair. The advent of computer microprocessors for power base wheelchairs

Chapter One: Getting to Know Your Wheels

has enabled the creation of control mechanisms for the users to control front-wheel, rear-wheel or mid-wheel drive chairs.

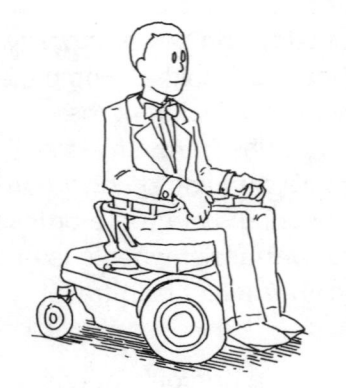

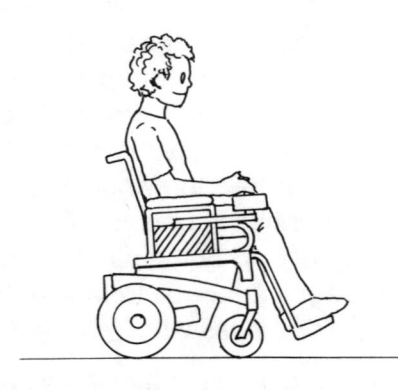

A typical front-wheel drive chair.

A typical rear-wheel drive chair.

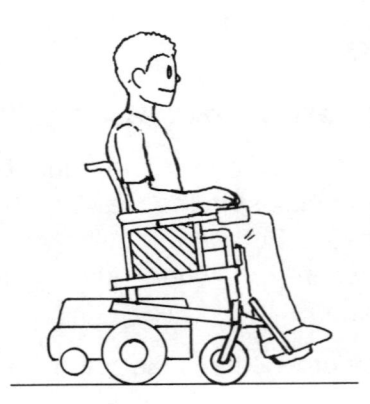

A typical mid-wheel drive chair.

The location of the drive wheel impacts the way the wheelchair handles and how it is steered. In a front-wheel drive chair, the mass of the wheelchair is behind the drive wheels. When the wheelchair slows down, there is a tendency for it to turn around backward. This is prevented by the controller, which keeps the wheelchair tracking straight by carefully monitoring the position of the front wheels. Front-wheel drive chairs have good traction going downhill, but can lose traction over sandy or slippery surfaces when going uphill, with the drive wheels pulling the chair forward.

The rear-wheel drive chair has the same difficulty with driving backward. When decelerating after driving backward, the wheelchair tends to try and turn. Rear-wheel drive chairs have better traction going uphill than they do going downhill.

Mid-wheel drive chairs have the potential for better traction than either front-wheel or rear-wheel drive chairs, because the drive wheels are located directly under the user's center of mass, putting maximum traction on the drive wheels. In a mid-wheel drive chair, the user has to get used to tipping back onto their small anti-tip wheels when going up a hill or during rapid acceleration. Mid-wheel drive powered wheelchairs may also be easier to maneuver in tight environments than either front-wheel or rear-wheel drive wheelchairs.

Section 1.3

Specifying the Seating Components and Control Input Device

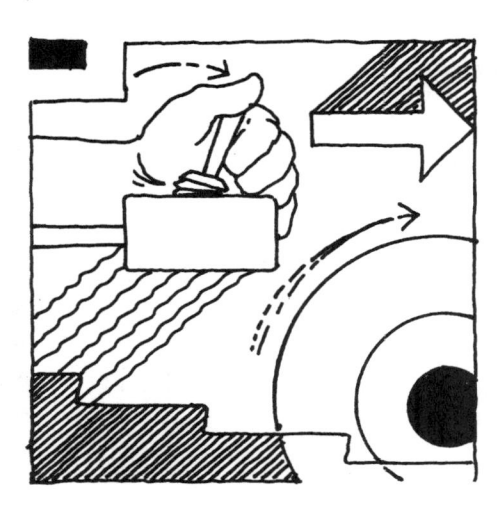

Selecting and Ordering Your Powered Wheelchair

This section of the book has limited information pertaining to the selection and ordering of your wheelchair. For more detailed and specific information on the proper selection and ordering of your powered wheelchair, we recommend that you consult *A Guide to Wheelchair Selection: How to Use the ANSI/RESNA Wheelchair Standards to Buy a Wheelchair* (see Appendix C for ordering information). That book reviews how to consider the performance information disclosed by the ANSI/RESNA wheelchair standards when selecting a powered wheelchair. This section of the book will briefly review the determination of the seat width and depth, back height, and the selection of accessories such as head support, arm supports, joysticks, lap belt, lateral supports, etc. Ideally, you will want to work with a RESNA certified Assistive Technology Practitioner (ATP) or Supplier (ATS) prior to making a purchase.

Seating Dimensions and Components

Seat width

Your wheelchair seat should be as narrow as possible without touching your hip bones. If the seat is too narrow, the pressure on bony hip prominences could cause a pressure ulcer. If the seat is too wide, it might cause you to lean more to one side, which could lead to the development of a spinal deformity. There should be about half an inch of space on either side of your thighs. The space gives you a little room to move and tuck in your clothing.

On most powered wheelchairs, the power base is the widest part of the wheelchair. If the seating system is the widest part of the wheelchair, the seat width can affect the overall width of the wheelchair. Power base wheelchairs usually allow for greater adjustment in seat width without widening the overall width of the wheelchair, as the seat structure is separate from the power base.

Transportable chairs have the seating surface as an integral part of the powered wheelchair. There are more limited options for altering the size or style of seating in these systems.

Chapter One: Getting to Know Your Wheels

This seat is too narrow.

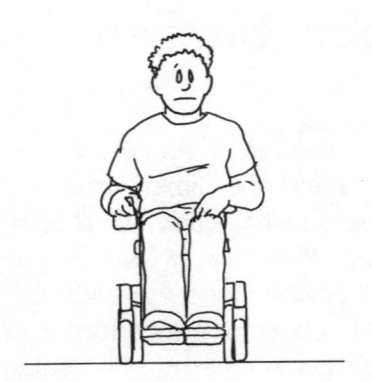

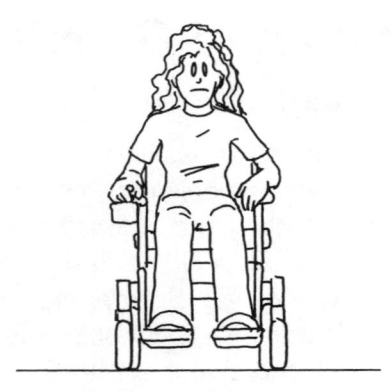

This seat is too wide.

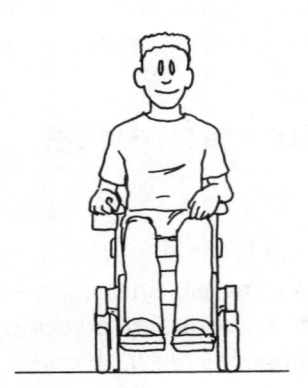

This seat is just right.

Seat depth

The right seat depth is essential for providing the proper amount of support under your thighs. If the seat is too deep, you will be unable to move all the way against the back support, and you will end up slouching back. A seat that is too deep can cause pressure on the backs of your knees and calves. This could interfere with circulation to your legs. If the seat is too shallow, you will experience more pressure on your sitting area, and you could develop pressure ulcers.

The correct seat depth typically permits one inch of space between the front edge of the cushion and the back of the knee. The space needed may be larger if you regularly use your hands to lift your legs.

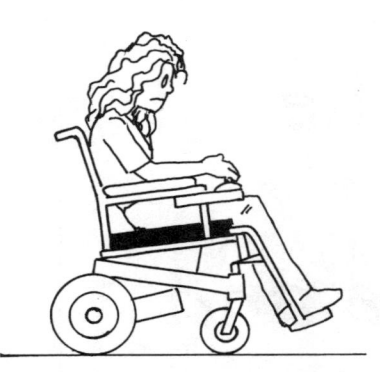

This seat is too long, causing the user to slouch.

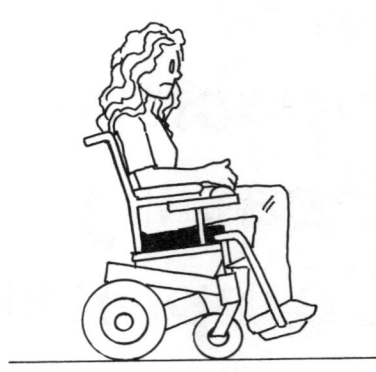

This seat is too short. The front part of the thighs are not supported.

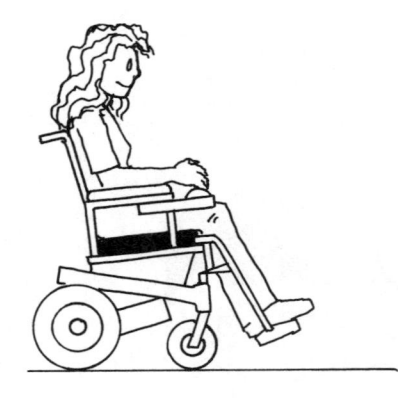

This seat is just the right depth.

If the seat upholstery or seat depth is too long:
- Talk to a seating specialist about shortening the upholstery or inserting a shorter solid seat in place of the upholstery.
- Insert a thicker back support, which will support your back further forward in your seat and shorten the overall seat depth.

If only the seat cushion is too long:
- Get a shorter cushion or modify the rear corners of the so it fits farther back on the seat.
- Slide the cushion back. Sometimes the cushion will slide under the back support. Make sure your buttocks are still positioned correctly on the cushion. Most pressure management cushions cannot be repositioned in this manner since the user must sit on the correct part of the cushion to optimize pressure distribution.

If the seat depth is too short:
- Move the back support back. This will allow you to slide farther back in your wheelchair, lengthening the seat depth and making room for a longer cushion.
- Use a longer seat cushion supported over the front edge of the seat by a firm board, a longer solid seat insert, or a sheet of stiff plastic.

If the seat cushion is too short:
- Get a longer cushion. On a chair with a solid seat base, an extension may be added to the front of a seat cushion.
- On a chair with sling upholstery, a sheet of flexible plastic can be put inside the seat cushion cover, beneath the cushion. This will help support a longer seat cushion that extends forward off of the seat upholstery.

Seat surface height

Your wheelchair seat must be high enough to accommodate the length of your lower legs with your feet on the foot supports. The seat should be high enough for your foot supports to clear obstacles and low enough for your knees to fit under tables. According to the Americans with Disabilities Act Accessibility Guidelines, standard tables or counters should have knee clearance spaces at least 27 inches high, 30 inches wide, and 19 inches deep. To determine the correct seat surface height:

- Sit on your seat cushion in your wheelchair with the foot supports properly adjusted.
- Make sure there is a minimum of 2 inches of clearance under your foot supports to maneuver safely outdoors. If your foot supports are too low, they will catch on the ground when going through curb ramps and will catch on small step transitions and curbs.
- Measure the vertical distance form the floor to the top of the seat surface.

If your legs are long, you might have to compromise between sitting comfort and foot support clearance. In a powered chair, the ground clearance of your footplate is a safety consideration. It is, therefore, more important for your wheelchair to fit properly and be able to clear obstacles with your footrests than to be able to roll under tables.

Because the motor and batteries are located beneath the seat in powered wheelchairs, you may not be able to order the seat surface height low enough to get as much knee clearance as you would like. You may be forced to drive up to tables and counters from the side to avoid hitting your knees on the edge.

Another important issue on table access is joystick clearance. If you can order a swing-away joystick, this will allow you to move the joystick off to the side to enable you to pull up closer to a table. You must be very cautious to avoid getting your joystick caught beneath the table, as this can cause a serious incident if the joystick cannot return to the off position. This situation has caused many powered wheelchairs to unintentionally rearrange all of the tables in a meeting room, scattering papers, people and causing injuries to wheelchair users and their meeting table companions.

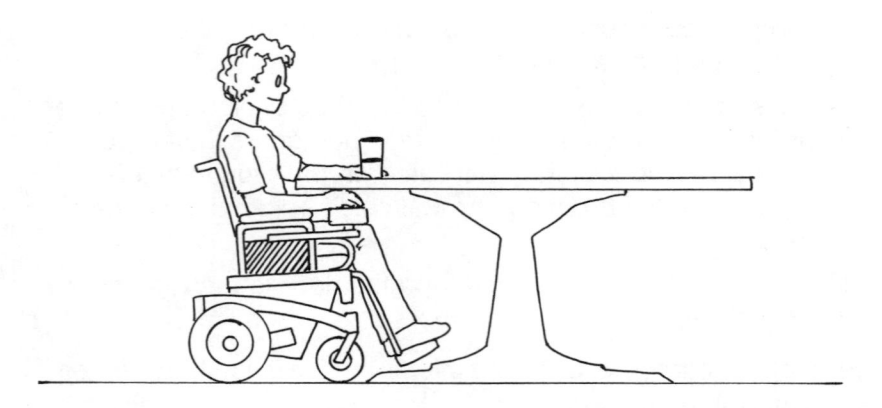

This person has enough knee and joystick clearance.

Back support height and angle

The back support height should be just high enough so that it does not interfere with shoulder or arm movements yet provides support to your back while in the chair. Try sitting in and driving wheelchairs with different back heights to determine the appropriate back height that allows you the movement and the support you need.

You may wish to look at a chair with an adjustable back angle to achieve the desired seat to back angle that is comfortable for you.

Arm supports

You will often need to specify the arm support style. Arm supports are typically available in desk or full length styles. The ability to adjust the height of the arm support is very important for good shoulder and arm positioning. Arm supports typically have standard pads, but there are many optional accessory pads with contours on the side and on the back to help maintain your arm position on the arm support. It is critical for control of your wheelchair to have good positioning of the arm that operates the chair. Your elbows should be slightly forward of your shoulders when your arms are resting on the arm supports. Straps can also be attached to the arm support pad to maintain your arm position for outdoor mobility.

Head support

A head support can help hold your head up when you are in your powered wheelchair or provide a support to help eliminate fatigue. Obstacles, rough terrain, sudden acceleration, or sharp maneuvering can make it difficult for you to support your head and may make it desirable to use a head support. Many wheelchair users do not like the look of having a head support on their wheelchair. The head support sticks up above the back of the wheelchair, potentially making the transport in and out of a vehicle more difficult.

All users who sit in their wheelchairs while riding in vehicles should use a head support to reduce the likelihood of whiplash injuries in the event of abrupt stops and starts. However, be aware that very few head supports have been tested for crashworthiness and are generally not designed to withstand the high impact forces that would occur in a crash situation.

Powered seating

Powered seating systems are an available option if you do not have the ability to do weight shifts while you are sitting in your wheelchair. Wheelchairs with powered seating systems are available that tilt your entire body back, recline the back, or both, while you are still in the chair. Reclining or tilting back reduces the pressure under your buttocks.

Lap trays

Lap trays are important to some people and are another accessory generally available and often used on powered chairs. Lap trays are a critical item for some wheelchair users. The tray becomes one's personal workspace for eating, reading or perhaps for operating a laptop computer or personal communication device. Lap trays have to be removable for transfers and need to be solid enough to support the weight of a variety of personal items.

Lap belts

A lap belt is an accessory that is provided with most powered wheelchairs. It is designed to keep you in your chair if you come to an abrupt stop, such as when your foot support contacts the bottom of a curb ramp, launching your upper body forward. Lap belts are rarely designed or intended to be used as seat belts in motor vehicles. Only if the wheelchair and lap belt have been tested as a system and meet the transportable wheelchair test standards should you expect your wheelchair lap belt combination to be safe for transport. Otherwise, you will need to use an additional seat belt attached to the vehicle. In either case, the restraint system that attaches from the vehicle to your wheelchair should be a tested, forward-facing system.

Trunk and lateral supports

To maintain better trunk stability, you may want to consider extended lateral supports and/or a chest strap. A chest strap is a strap that goes across the chest and underneath the arms. An over-the-shoulder style chest support can offer the same advantages if you prefer this type of strap.

Joystick Type

This book focuses on techniques for people who can operate a joystick with their hand to control their powered wheelchair. Many people are unable to use hand-operated joysticks and require alternate control systems for their wheelchairs. A few common alternate controls are described here. If you want more information about these and other alternate controls, contact your wheelchair supplier or other rehabilitation professional before ordering.

Joystick options

Most powered wheelchairs are only sold with one joystick option, which can usually be set up either on the left or right hand side of the chair. Look for positioning hardware that allows final adjustment of the joystick position relative to the arm supports. Some users may want to be able to rotate the joystick control inward about the vertical axis.

Long throw vs. short throw

Look at the amount of joystick movement from full forward to full reverse on different wheelchair models. If you only have a small amount of hand movement, or if your strength prevents you from pushing the joystick through its full range of motion, you may choose a **short throw** option.

- A short throw option allows the same range of speed (from zero to maximum speed) as a joystick operating in full throw, by moving the joystick approximately half the distance.
- A short throw option allows a person with weakness in their hand or arm to achieve maximum speed.
- Good fine motor coordination is necessary to operate a short throw joystick successfully.

Swing-away joystick mount

On many chairs the joystick mounting can be ordered to retract or swing away to the side to allow you to pull your wheelchair closer to a table top. A detent, or latch, often holds the joystick in the swing-away or driving position.

Alternate Controls

Alternative joystick

Some people can control their wheelchair with a joystick operated by another part of the body other than the hand. Joysticks can be mounted for use with your foot, elbow, arm, chin, or even behind your head. Make sure the mounting is secure but moves out of the way as needed for transfers. An alternate joystick knob, such as a tennis ball or a suction cup, may also be used.

Sip and puff

An air switch can be attached to a tube so the user can sip or blow into a pair of tubes to make the chair move. Usually the person needs to have at least four different capabilities for this type of control: soft and hard sip, and soft and hard puff. These different inputs control movement in the left, right, forward, and backward directions.

Multiple switches or wafer board

Many types of switches are available. These switches can be pressed in a variety of ways, including using the fingers and elbows. Usually at least three switches are needed: one for forward and reverse, one for turning left and right, and one for stopping. Typically, the switches are mounted on a single board. There may be a ridge or a space between the switches so the wrong switch is not easily activated.

Head controls

Single switches can be mounted on a head support or other armature, allowing the operator to use head movements to control the wheelchair.

Proximity switch

A proximity switch can be used to monitor the position of the head. The wheelchair can be driven by moving the position of the head left or right to turn, forward to go straight ahead, etc.

Kill or safety switch

A separate power switch can be used to turn off the chair in an emergency and is often used or required with some alternative controls.

Section 1.4

Seating Setup and Wheel Adjustments

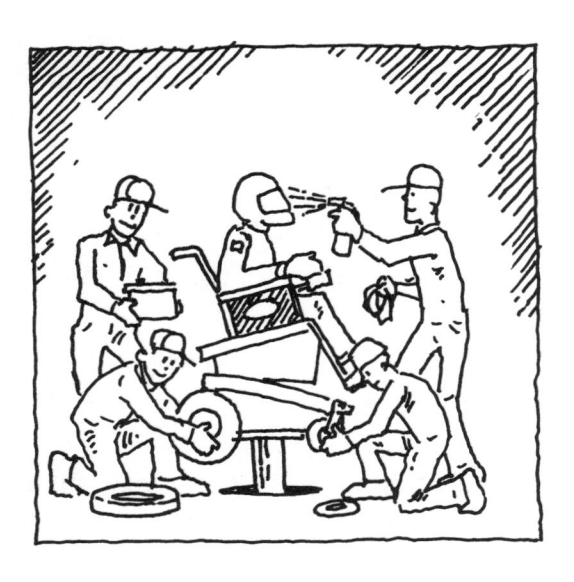

One change to your wheelchair usually affects the fit of all the other components, so be prepared to spend a fair amount of time setting up the seating and positioning within your wheelchair. Ideally, when adjusting your wheelchair, you should enlist the help of an assistive technology practitioner or supplier certified by RESNA (Rehabilitation Engineering and Assistive Technology Society of North America).

After each adjustment, test drive the wheelchair with assistance on ramps, different surfaces, and side slopes to make sure your mobility needs have been met. This can be done by driving the wheelchair onto a sloped surface or by physically tipping the wheelchair to its balance point in various directions. Extreme caution should be exercised using the help of multiple assistants. If your seating system is adjustable, the stability of your chair should also be checked with the seating system in all of its extreme positions.

Whenever you alter the setup of your wheelchair, check your forward, side-to-side, and rear stability with a spotter to make sure your wheelchair performs the way you would like.

The set up and adjustment of your wheelchair is a topic worthy of an entire book. There are many adjustments which you will probably refine over many years; others you will want to make throughout each day.

Seat Surface Angle Adjustment

The seat surface angle can be adjusted on some wheelchairs. A forward sloping seat might cause you to slide forward. Raising the front edge of the seat creates a "bucket" between the back support and seat and closes the seat-to-back angle. If the seat back is reclined at the same time the front of the seat is tipped upward, and the seat-to-back angle stays the same, this is called "tilt-in-space."

Several powered wheelchair frames allow seat angle adjustments. If the chair frame itself does not adjust, you can still adjust the seat surface angle by:

- Adding a wedge to the seat base beneath the seat cushion
- Purchasing a cushion that will angle the seat surface
- Adding a solid seat with angle adjustable hardware

Chapter One: Getting to Know Your Wheels

Back Angle Adjustment

Your back support angle should provide a comfortable sitting posture while you are upright in the chair. The back angle should not cause you to curl your shoulders, hold your head forward for balance, or cause you to slide out of your seat.

The angle formed by the seat and the back support is called the seat-to-back angle. A seat-to-back angle greater than 90 degrees is often referred to as an "open angle," while an angle smaller than 90 degrees is referred to as a "closed angle." An open angle lets you use gravity to help balance your trunk. People with high spinal cord injuries who cannot flex well at the hips often use an open seat-to-back angle. However, an open angle can cause people to slide down in their chairs. If you have the flexibility, a closed angle cradles the body in the curve of the seat, holding you in place. A more open or closed angle can often reduce spasticity.

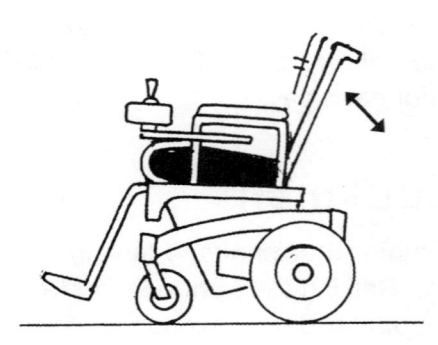

This powered wheelchair has an electrically powered reclining back support.

Drive Wheel Position Adjustment

Though less critical than on manual wheelchairs, the distribution of weight carried between the drive wheels and the casters on a powered chair will influence the driving performance of the chair. Due to the weight of a powered chair, when attempting to traverse soft terrain like gravel or sand, the chair will tend to sink and the casters will get stuck.

When negotiating low obstacles, for example small curbs, the location of the drive wheels (front, mid, or rear) can make a difference. On a few powered wheelchairs, the actual mounting position of the drive wheels on the frame can be adjusted. Alternatively, some manufacturers allow for adjustment of the seat frame on the power base. Moving the entire seat forward or backward on the power base has the same effect as moving the drive wheel mounting position – to redistribute the weight between the drive wheels and the casters.

Front-Wheel Drive – For the most part, the drive wheels on front-wheel drive chairs have a fixed mounting position on the frame. Frequently, the batteries will be positioned on the chair in such a way as to evenly distribute the weight on the frame, getting as much weight forward as possible. Because the casters are in the rear, one advantage to front-wheel drive chairs is the ability for you to just drive forward over obstacles. The larger drive wheels mounted in the front will not get "hung up," but rather will drive right up and over an obstacle.

Mid-Wheel Drive – This style of chair is available in a wide number of configurations. If you are interested in a mid-wheel drive style chair, it is important to test drive the particular wheelchair model to understand what effect the setup of drive wheels and casters will have on the drive performance of the chair. The first thing to look at is the actual position of the drive wheel on the frame. There is some variation among manufacturers as to where the drive wheels are mounted to the power base, relative to the seat:

- Directly under the seat
- Slightly behind the mid-point of the seat (though forward of the back posts)

Check with your supplier or the manufacturer to determine if the position of the seat or the drive wheel can be adjusted slightly forward or backward.

A "true" mid-wheel driving wheel location may increase the "rocking" of the chair when you rapidly speed-up or come to a quick stop. If you look carefully, some mid-wheel drive chairs are actually six-wheeled chairs, with two drive wheels and four stabilizing wheels (usually two casters in front and two large anti-tip wheels in the rear).

Rear-Wheel Drive – Rear-wheel drive chairs most often have a fixed drive wheel mount. The position of the batteries and your weight when sitting in the chair naturally tend to increase the load on the rear wheels. In many rear-wheel drive chairs, the actual mounting of the drive wheels is behind the backpost of the seat (placing your center of gravity in front of the wheels). This rear placement of the drive wheel makes for a very stable configuration that is more difficult to "pop a wheelie" (lifting the front casters off the ground). A very stable configuration may give you security when negotiating ramps and inclines, but will make negotiating small obstacles very difficult.

Changing the drive wheel position or the position of the seat on the frame is a "heavy duty" adjustment and most often should be done by a qualified wheelchair service technician.

Arm Support Height Adjustment

The arm support should be adjusted so the arms are not pulling down on the shoulders. Your elbows should be slightly forward of your shoulders when your arms are resting on the arm supports. The front-to-back position of the arm supports should allow the upper arm to slope forward slightly. Some people like to be able to pull their elbows back for stability on non-level surfaces. If your joystick is mounted on the arm support of the wheelchair, make sure you can reach it easily. When adjusting the arm support height on a wheelchair with power recline, make sure the arm support does not interfere with moving the back support from the completely reclined to fully upright position.

Caster Adjustments

Mounting adjustments

Your casters should be mounted on the frame so they are perpendicular to the ground. If they are not, your front casters may become afflicted with "shopping cart syndrome" and flutter when you drive your chair. This may also make it difficult to turn your wheelchair or change direction. Use a carpenter's square to verify that the caster housing is perpendicular to the ground.

Height and suspension adjustments

Due to the tendency of a mid-wheel drive chair to "rock," there are smaller wheels mounted on the front and the back of the chair. Look carefully at these wheels. In most cases, one set will be allowed to swivel and will function as casters. The second set are fixed and will function as anti-tip devices. The position of the "caster wheels" and the "anti-tipper wheels" may be at the front or rear, depending on the specific wheelchair design.

Frequently, the "anti-tipper wheels" will have these adjustments:
- Height off the ground
- Tension of suspension

Height – The position of the anti-tip wheels off the ground will affect the amount of rocking you feel when you either accelerate rapidly or come to a quick stop. The closer the wheels are to the ground, the less rocking you will experience. However, the closer the wheels are to the ground, the greater the likelihood will be of getting "hung-up." If the anti-tipper wheels are too close to the ground, when you drive off of a small threshold or through a curb ramp, you run the risk of having all the "little" wheels being on the ground, with the drive wheels being "suspended" in the air. With no drive wheels contacting the ground, you are stuck!

Suspension – In an attempt to reduce the likelihood of getting hung-up and to smooth out the "rocking" sensation, some models have suspension in the anti-tipper wheels. The spring in the suspension may be adjustable to match your weight and driving style. Other power base wheelchairs have suspension on the casters and the main drive wheels.

Much like any adjustment to the drive wheel position, changing the height or tension of the anti-tipper wheels is a "heavy-duty" adjustment. Working with a trained wheelchair technician can facilitate getting the adjustments made to meet your driving style.

Foot Support Adjustment

Adjust your foot supports after you have your seat cushion, back support, and other positioning aids in place. Don't forget to put your shoes on; sole height affects your leg positioning. Make sure you are seated upright against the back of the chair. When adjusting the foot supports, make sure you have:

- A minimum clearance of 2 inches underneath the foot plates
- Clearance for your knees under desks and tables

If you do not have enough foot or knee clearance, you might need to readjust your seat height. If your feet are supported at the correct height by your foot supports, your thighs should rest in a balanced manner on your cushion. Foot supports that are too high can lead to little or no weight under the thighs and excessive weight under your sitting bones, the ischial tuberosities. You might need to compromise on your knee height to get the desired weight distribution on the seat cushion.

If your knees will not fit under a table, you can slip coasters or wooden blocks under the table legs to raise the table up higher. At a restaurant, it is possible to turn small plates upside down and slide them underneath each of the table legs. Make sure the table is secure and will not slip off the leg props.

Seat Height Adjustment

To increase the foot support to ground clearance (raise yourself higher off the ground), you can adjust the seat up. Alternatively, you can increase the seat cushion thickness by adding a layer of stiff foam or a solid insert under the seat cushion. If all of the wheels are vertically adjustable it may be possible to move all of the wheels lower to raise the seat height, or to raise all of the wheels to lower the seat height.

To lower your knee height and decrease ground clearance (lower yourself closer to the ground), you could decrease the thickness of the seat cushion only if appropriate.

Sometimes you can push your knees down as you pull forward underneath the table and your knees can spring back up under the table. If you try this, be sure that there is not too much pressure on the top of your legs from the edge of the table.

Swing-away foot supports permit you to get under some obstacles because one or both foot supports can be removed, allowing the feet to dangle and the knees to drop lower for maneuvering in tight quarters. If you do this, you will need to be very careful backing up from underneath the table. The casters can swing around and catch on your feet, potentially causing injury.

Section 1.5

Joystick Setup, Adjustments and Operation

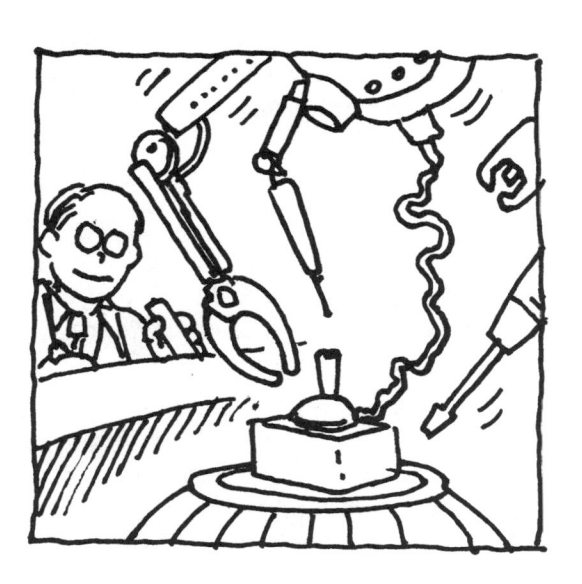

The joystick is the command center of your wheelchair. It typically consists of a control shaft that ends in a ball socket. The joystick can be moved in any direction within the rectangular housing. The joystick functions as steering wheel, accelerator and brake – all in one. In most cases, pushing the joystick in a particular direction will drive the wheelchair in that direction. Like the accelerator of a car, the farther you push the joystick from the neutral position, the faster the wheelchair will move. Many wheelchair models allow you to set the maximum forward, reverse, and turning speeds.

Joystick Positioning

The position of the joystick is a matter of personal preference. Some people find it easier to keep their joystick directly in front of the arm support, others prefer to position it inside or outside of the arm support. All these positions can be arranged for either left or right hand control. Keep in mind that some joystick positions, particularly forward of the arm support, may prevent you from getting under tables. If you cannot use your hands to move the joystick and require an alternate control method, contact your wheelchair supplier and/or rehab professional for help. Alternate controls are described briefly in Section 1.3.

Helpful Hints

If you find that your joystick box tends to hit the edge of tables, you might want to order a swing-away or retractable joystick mount. This will allow you to swing away, pivot or retract the controls to the side so that you can get closer to the table.

Joystick Handles

Depending on your gripping and holding abilities, you may want to select a different shape or size of joystick handle. If someone does not have fine motor control in their fingertips, an alternative control knob allowing open palm use will be desired. If your hand is weak or has poor control, choose a control knob that fits underneath your hand securely.

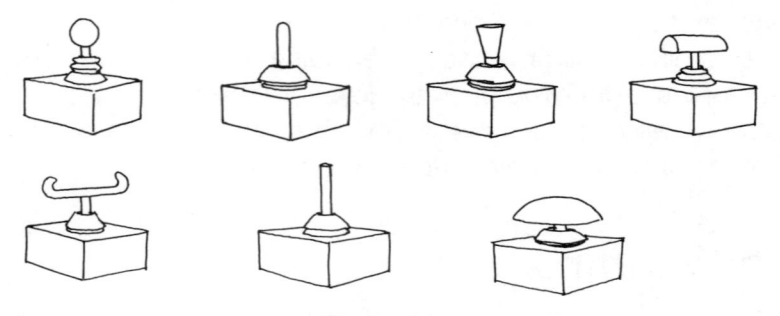

A variety of joystick handles are available.

You might also need to use a splint along with a joystick handle to control your wheelchair.

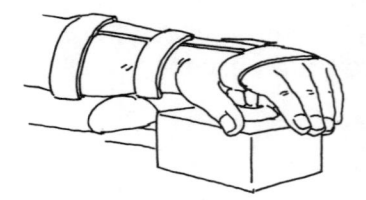

A hand splint may help you hold on to the joystick.

Things to consider when experimenting with the joystick position:

- Make sure you can operate the joystick in all directions, that the on/off control is easily activated and that the speed control can be adjusted.
- Can you operate the on/off switch without accidentally hitting the joystick?
- Can you operate the joystick without accidentally hitting the on/off or other switches?
- Be aware that switches can sometimes be repositioned by the manufacturer.

- A joystick mounting bracket may be available that allows the joystick to swing out of the way for clearance under tables and other low surfaces.
- The joystick does not necessarily need to be positioned so that a forward push causes the chair to move forward. If your arm is angled in, you might want to push the joystick at a diagonal in order for the wheelchair to go forward.
- Experimentation with joystick positioning can be accomplished with an adjustable support such as the Magic Arm™ by Bogen.
- Once you have identified the joystick position that works best for you, have it mounted permanently in its final position. Your wheelchair supplier should do this for you.

Dealer Programmable Drive Performance Adjustments

The following parameters, which affect the drive performance of the chair, can often be adjusted using a special programmer available from the dealer.

Not all powered wheelchairs have these adjustment options. Many of these adjustments may need to be made by your equipment supplier to maintain the warranty or because the adjustments require special programmers and expertise. Refer to your owner's manual for more details.

Maximum forward speed

- The maximum forward speed is how fast the wheelchair can go when you push the joystick all the way forward. The maximum speed varies from chair to chair. Your top speed can usually be programmed as you desire.
- Many wheelchairs have multiple driving modes that can be programmed separately, such as Drive A and B, Indoor and Outdoor, or Low, Medium and High. Once each option is programmed, you can select one of several maximum forward speed settings. Many models that allow for several settings to

be programmed to handle different driving conditions, such as crowded versus open spaces or rough versus smooth surfaces, allow a lot of versatility.

Maximum reverse speed

- The maximum reverse speed is how fast the wheelchair can go when you push the joystick all the way backward.
- Some wheelchairs allow a maximum reverse speed to be programmed independently of the maximum forward speed.
- Sometimes maximum reverse speed is programmed to be a percentage of maximum forward speed. For instance, if the manufacturer sets the maximum reverse speed at 50% and you set the maximum forward speed at 4 miles per hour, the fastest you will be able to go in reverse is 2 miles per hour.

Maximum turning rate

- The maximum turning rate is how fast you can turn in a circle.
- Some wheelchair manufacturers program the maximum turning rate as a percentage of the maximum forward speed.

Turning acceleration

- The turning acceleration rate is how quickly you can increase the turning speed up to the maximum turning rate.
- If the turning acceleration is programmed too high, the chair may fishtail in and out of turns and your body may be thrown from side to side. Through programming, you can often reduce the acceleration rate if you have problems with directional control.

Forward and reverse acceleration

- The overall maximum acceleration rate is how quickly you can increase your speed to the maximum forward and reverse speeds.
- Both forward and reverse acceleration are often programmed separately or by the overall maximum acceleration rate.

- A high acceleration rate will result in very responsive controls.
- If you have poor trunk or head control, reducing the acceleration rate may give you a more comfortable ride.
- On some wheelchairs, a high acceleration rate can cause the front wheels to lift off the ground in a wheelie.

Forward and reverse deceleration

- The overall **maximum deceleration rate** is how quickly you can slow down from the maximum forward speed or maximum reverse speed.
- Maximum deceleration will cause the chair to stop almost immediately.
- If you do not have good trunk or head control, a quick stop may cause you to fall forward or whip your head and neck around. Reducing the maximum deceleration may give you a more comfortable ride.
- On the other hand, **minimum deceleration** will increase the braking distance, or the distance the chair will travel before coming to a complete stop.
- There may be separate programmability for forward and reverse deceleration, or there may be a deceleration setting that controls deceleration for both forward and reverse.

Turning deceleration

- The turning deceleration rate is how quickly your turning rate will decrease when you let go of the joystick.
- If the turning deceleration rate is set too high, your upper body may be thrown to the side as a turning chair comes to a stop.

Overall sensitivity or tremor dampening

- An overall sensitivity rating allows compensation for tremor or spasticity in the joystick input control. It filters out movements caused by tremor or spasticity.
- Not all wheelchairs allow programming of sensitivity.

Reversal of Controls

For some wheelchair riders it is very difficult to hold the joystick pushed forward, but possible to hold it back. It is possible with some programmable controllers to reverse the joystick controls such that pulling back causes the wheelchair to go forward. This should not be accomplished by turning the joystick around backward, because this would also switch the left and right directional controls. Moving the joystick to the left or right should cause the wheelchair to turn in that direction.

User Adjustable Settings and Joystick Operations

There are usually some settings on your controller that permit you to adjust certain aspects of your wheelchair performance throughout the day. You may wish to make adjustments depending on where you are using the chair. Some adjustments may require reprogramming of the controller by the dealer. Other adjustments may not be possible at all.

Not all powered wheelchairs have these user accessible adjustment options. Some of these adjustments may need to be made by your equipment supplier to maintain the warranty or because the adjustments require special tools and expertise. Refer to your owner's manual for more details.

Speed (velocity)

As noted earlier, a proportional joystick lets you control speed and direction at the same time. How *far* you move the stick from the center will determine how *fast* the chair will travel, much like the gas pedal on a car. You control the speed of the chair by adjusting the position of the stick closer or further away from the center.

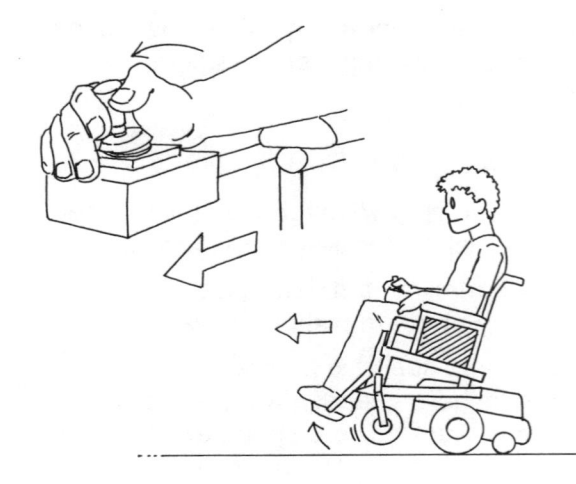

Pushing your joystick all the way forward will make the wheelchair accelerate forward to maximum speed.

Acceleration and deceleration

Acceleration is the drive parameter which reflects the "pick-up" of the chair or how quickly the chair achieves top speed after you place the joystick at the "full throw" position. Two chairs can be set up with the same top speed and have very different acceleration rates. Eventually, both chairs will be traveling at the same speed, but the chair with the slower acceleration will have "ramped up" to that speed more slowly. The rate of acceleration needs to be programmed into the chair by an authorized assistive technology dealer or supplier.

If your wheelchair lurches as you drive along, consider reducing the acceleration and/or deceleration settings. This allows you to adjust how quickly the wheelchair will pick up speed or come to a stop. Once you set these, you should be able to maintain maximum speed without losing your balance and remain in a speed range that is comfortable for you. If you are still uncomfortable with the performance of the chair, you may want to reduce the maximum forward and reverse speed.

If you wish to check your deceleration setting, drive your wheelchair toward a line on the ground at normal cruising speed and stop the wheelchair just as you cross the line. Measure the distance it took to come to a stop. Now try adjusting the deceleration and repeat the stopping procedure.

Repeat the same adjustments for turning if you lose your balance or are uncomfortable with how fast you turn. Read your owner's manual to determine what you can adjust on your own and work with your supplier to customize these settings to reflect your driving preferences and local terrain.

Methods of deceleration (stopping)

- **Let go of the joystick.** The chair may roll before coming to a stop.
- Sometimes, you can **pull backward on the joystick** (into reverse) to stop more quickly than if you let go of the joystick. Prior to the existence of digital controllers, manufacturers did NOT recommend this technique because it could permanently damage components on wheelchairs with non-digital electronics.
- **Emergency stopping (power off).** If the wheelchair is moving erratically, or not moving in the intended direction due to a controller malfunction, turn off the power. The emergency "fail safe" brakes will automatically be applied and bring you to an abrupt stop. Have your wheelchair set up so you can easily reach the on/off or "kill" switch in case you need to do this in an emergency. Practice this emergency stop so you can see what it feels like. A lap belt, chest strap and/or a spotter may be needed so you do not lose your balance or fall from the chair while practicing.

Steering

- Use small movements of the joystick to the left or right to make minor adjustments to your course while driving the wheelchair forward.
- To make a sharp, fast turn, move the joystick directly from the center to the left or right.
- Many wheelchairs have a tendency to veer to one side. Veering can occur for many reasons, such as when the motor on one side of your chair is less efficient, if one tire is low on air, if you have a belt-driven wheelchair and one belt is more worn or stretched than the other, or when you drive on a cross slope. Correct veering with small movements of the joystick. Some chairs also have a veer adjustment.

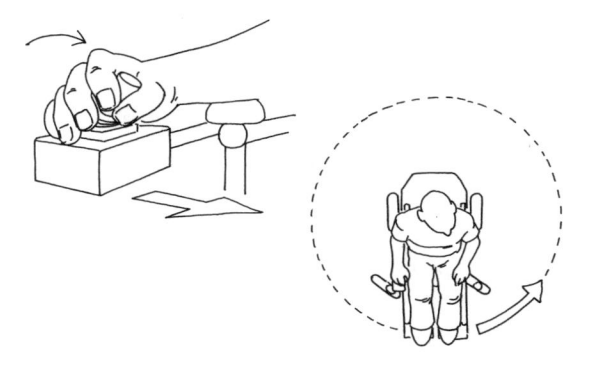

Push your joystick to the side to make a sharp turn.

Cruise control

Some powered wheelchairs have a cruise control or latch option. When cruise control is on, your chair will continue to travel forward at a set speed without requiring you to hold the joystick forward. When the cruise control is off, you will have to push the joystick to control the wheelchair. With the wheelchair in "cruise," you should be able to use your joystick to make direction changes.

Cruise control is helpful if you fatigue easily and travel for long distances in the same direction. However, cruise control could be dangerous if there are obstacles you need to drive around or rough surfaces to cross.

If your wheelchair has cruise control, you need to have a kill switch or on/off switch to be able to immediately stop the wheelchair in case you are unable to move the drive control to stop.

Checking Your Stability with a Spotter

Once the seating system has been set up and adjusted, the joystick moved to a comfortable position, and the controller programmed, check the stability of the wheelchair system with a spotter. This will help you understand the limit of your wheelchair's stability. When performing any stability test, be sure the anti-tippers are in a functional position and that there is a spotter present. Anti-tippers are small wheels attached to the back or front of your wheelchair that prevent the wheelchair from tipping over. If possible, have the spotter hold the reset switch while walking alongside the wheelchair. In the event of an unsafe situation, the spotter can hold down the front end of the wheelchair or even shut off the power.

Check your stability on level surfaces

- Find a flat, wide-open surface such as an empty parking lot or basketball court.
- A spotter standing behind you should prevent the wheelchair from tipping over backward.
- Push the joystick forward to take off at maximum forward speed.
- Check to see if the front wheels pop up. Some people do not mind a wheelchair that performs this way, but front wheel popping could cause you to tip over backward in a conventional rear-wheel drive wheelchair when going up a steep ramp.
- Mid-wheel drive wheelchairs are designed to allow the front wheels to pop up in the air while the large anti-tip wheels contact the ground in the rear.
- Drive in reverse first and then immediately apply full power forward to see if the results are any different.

Check your stability going up ramps

- Find a standard ramp (see Section 3.5 for more information about ramps).
- A spotter standing behind you should prevent the wheelchair from tipping over backward.
- Accelerate forward at full speed.
- Check to see if the front wheels pop up. Some people do not mind a wheelchair that performs this way. Others may lose their trunk balance when this happens.

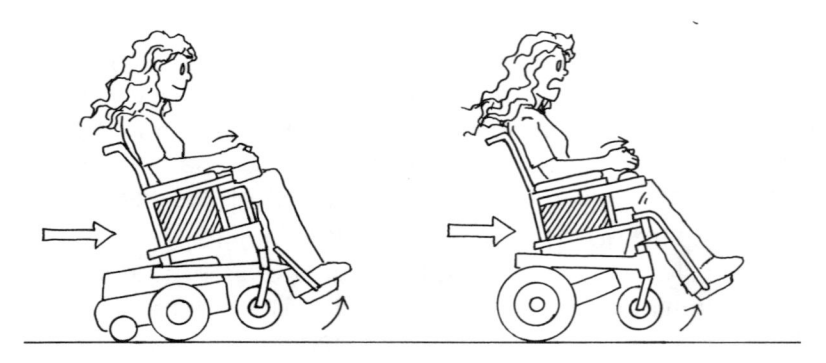

Sometimes the front wheels will pop up as you speed away.

Check your stability going down ramps

- A spotter standing next to you should be prepared to catch your upper body if you fall forward.
- Drive the wheelchair down a standard ramp at full speed.
- Release the joystick for maximum deceleration.
- If you fall too far forward, you may need to use a postural support, such as a chest or shoulder strap, or to reduce the maximum deceleration setting to prevent this from happening.

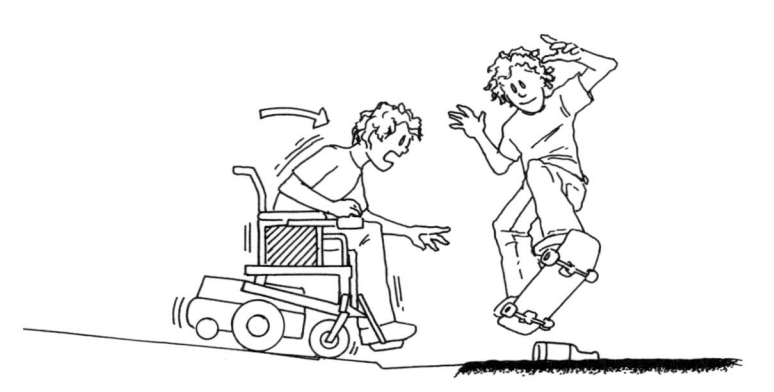

If you fall forward, a chest strap or other postural support can help keep you upright.

Check your stability as you turn

- Have a spotter follow along on the side opposite to the direction you are turning, prepared to catch you if you lose your balance.
- Perform a turn at maximum acceleration on a flat surface.
- Let go of the joystick for maximum deceleration.
- Check to see if you need any postural supports to avoid falling from side to side, or if you need to adjust the maximum turning acceleration rate. Chest or lap belts may also be appropriate.

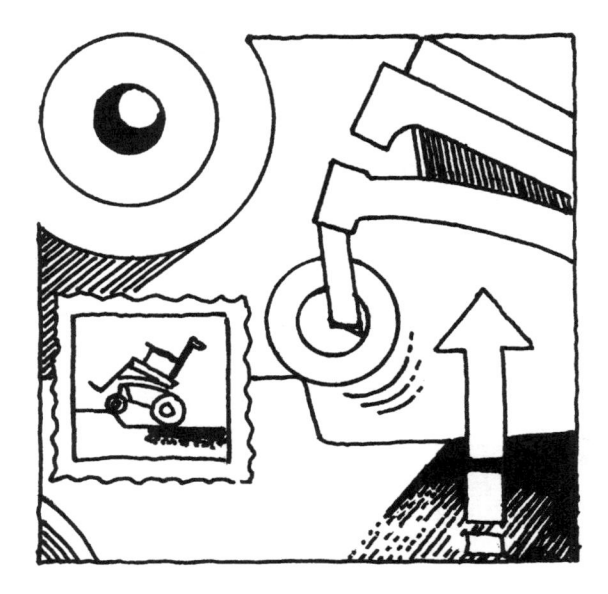

General Skills

CHAPTER 2

In this Chapter

2.1	Asking for Help	26
2.2	Learning Your Limits	30
2.3	Relieving Pressure	34
2.4	Reaching, Bending and Lifting	38
2.5	Main Wheel and Caster Management	41

Chapter 2 provides basic information on how powered wheelchairs work and how you can begin using yours as effectively as possible. The skills and techniques described in this guide are written for people operating a powered wheelchair with a hand-operated joystick. If you are unable to use a hand-operated joystick, many other types of wheelchair control options are available to provide you with independent mobility, some of which are covered in Chapter 1.

This guide does not cover the many different types of transfers that you need to know for wheelchair use. Physical or occupational therapists teach transfers from a wheelchair to bathtubs, toilets, beds and other areas. Only floor-to-wheelchair transfers, which are likely to be encountered in emergency situations, are discussed in Chapter 4 Emergency Skills.

Before practicing the maneuvers in this chapter, read the warnings on page xi to learn about the risks involved. Remember that for some wheelchair riders, falling may result in severe injury or death.

Chapter Two: General Skills

Section 2.1

Asking for Help

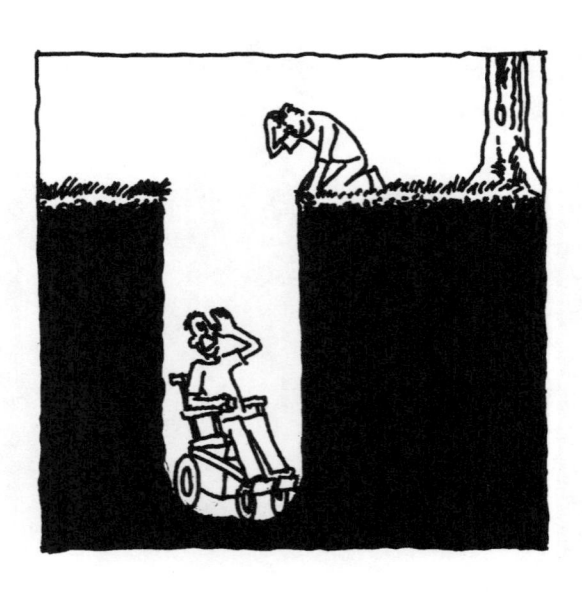

Access improvements for people with disabilities are being made every day. However, you will still encounter situations where you need help.

Everyone with or without a disability needs help now and then. The need for assistance will vary from situation to situation, and person to person. The hardest part for many people is knowing and understanding when they have reached their limits.

Defining "Assistance"

"Assistance" has many meanings. You may need to be lifted up stairs, helped over a loose gravel pathway, up a steep ramp, across a street, up or down a curb, over a railroad track, etc.

- **Independent Skills:** Independent skills are those things you can do without help.
- **Supervised/Assisted Skills:** Supervised/assisted skills are those things you are uncomfortable doing totally by yourself, but you can do partially. You might need occasional help or someone nearby "just in case." Being able to ask for help and being able to instruct others is very important.
- **Dependent Skills:** Dependent skills are those things you can only do with a lot of help.

Who Can Help?

The amount of help you need will depend on your present skills and abilities, as well as the task you need to accomplish. In some cases, you might want someone nearby because you are learning a new skill or you are just a bit unsure about the situation. At other times, you may be trying to get past an obstruction that you are unable to negotiate. This section gives you some pointers on working with different kinds of helpers, including spotters, assistants, personal care attendants or PCA's, family or friends, coworkers, acquaintances and strangers.

Spotter

A spotter is a person who stands nearby to help if you need it. Always use a spotter when learning a new skill, such as driving down a steep ramp, and when you are not confident in your ability to handle a situation alone. The spotter could help to prevent you from tipping or falling forward out of your wheelchair. It is up to you to decide when you are uncomfortable with a maneuver and would like to use a spotter. You might need more than one spotter when learning a new skill. It is also important to instruct your spotter(s) as to exactly how you need to be spotted. For example, going down a ramp you might ask a spotter to walk alongside of the wheelchair, ready to catch your upper body should you lose your balance in the forward direction.

Assistant

A spotter becomes an assistant when you know you will need help or will require more assistance than someone standing by offering an occasional hand. Assisting often involves pushing or lifting the wheelchair in some capacity (e.g., up a curb or threshold that is too high to cross independently). An assistant might also be required to perform other tasks, such as picking up things you drop or getting things you cannot reach. In many cases, an assistant is hired and trained by the wheelchair rider. These assistants are often referred to as personal care assistants (PCA's) and attendants.

Personal Care Assistant (PCA)

If you need help frequently or at regular times during the day, you may want to hire a personal care assistant. Some wheelchair users find it difficult to ask a family member or a friend to help because they feel they are burdening them. Relationships with family members or friends may become strained if they always feel responsible for helping you.

A potential advantage of a hired assistant is that the assistant can help you with personal tasks, such as bowel and bladder care, and is generally not as emotionally involved with you.

It is the job of a hired assistant to provide the help you need in a given situation. You can train your professional assistant to do things the way you want. If the arrangement does not work out, you also have the freedom to replace the PCA.

Family and friends

Family and friends with whom you spend most of your time will need to spot or assist you on some occasions. It can be valuable to rely on people you feel comfortable with when facing a difficult or challenging situation.

Do not assume that a family member or friend will always be comfortable helping you. Be sure to ask if they are willing to help. Make sure they know not to help you unless you request assistance. You probably have a good idea of which friends and family members you can trust as assistants based on your familiarity with their personalities.

Coworkers or acquaintances

Coworkers or friendly acquaintances can also make good assistants when you need help at work. If you are on good terms with a coworker, you may be comfortable casually asking for assistance (e.g., "Hi. Can you give me a push over this threshold?").

People you meet after your injury may be more comfortable with you as a wheelchair user than friends or family still making the adjustment to your new circumstances.

Strangers

When you are alone, situations may arise where you need the assistance of a stranger. For example, you may have dropped your car keys where you cannot reach them. In these cases, you may need to ask someone you do not know for help.

Alternatively, you may be out with a friend and find yourself in a situation where the assistance of a second person is necessary. For example, you may need an additional person to help lift the front end of your wheelchair up a curb.

How to Ask for Help

How you ask for help will vary from situation to situation. Ask for assistance in a way that allows the person to comfortably decline. You can practice asking for assistance with a companion acting as a stranger. This will help you learn how to ask strangers for assistance, as well as teach your companion to help only when asked. This type of practice also helps you learn how to instruct others to safely assist you.

Remember that there can be many valid reasons for people to decline to help you. Some people have disabilities that may not be visible, such as arthritis or heart disease, and they may be reluctant to disclose their condition to you. Other people's beliefs or customs may present a barrier to assisting you.

Gracefully accept refusals to help. After all, you don't want help from a person who feels uncomfortable with the task because their apprehension can increase the risk of injury for both of you.

Consider the following before asking a stranger for help:

- Do not ask for assistance from anyone you feel might be a threat.
- Consider the people around you and approach only those who look prepared to provide some physical assistance.
- Body size is not that critical when performing most assisting skills. Do not assume a smaller person is not strong enough to help you.

- Ask for assistance from people involved in activities similar to your own. For example, if you are shooting baskets in the park and lose the basketball in a bush, ask another ball player for assistance.
- If you enjoy challenging environments, such as hiking trails, remember that this type of environment attracts a lot of people who, like yourself, might be looking for an adventure. They may see helping you as yet another challenge and be very eager to assist.
- If there are few people around and you know you will need assistance soon (e.g., there is a curb around the corner), ask someone if they would be willing to follow you to the place where you will need help.
- Try "Do you mind giving me a hand up this curb?" or "Could you help me down this steep curb ramp? I can talk you through what I need you to do."

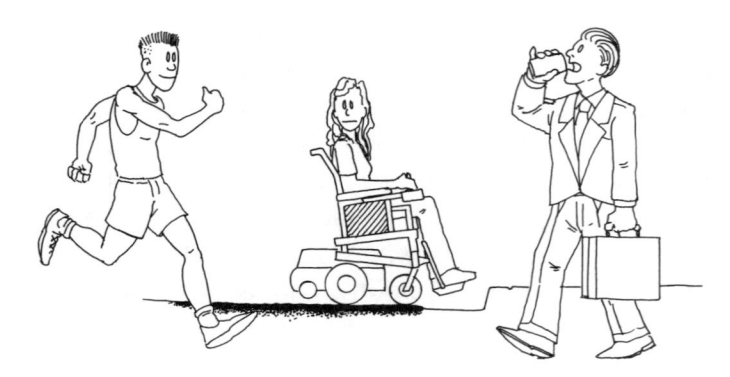

Observe the people around you and ask those who look ready and willing to assist.

Be clear and concise when giving instructions. Most of the skills in this book include instructions you can give an assistant.

- You are in charge. Instruct your assistant not to do anything unless you specifically ask.

- Read Section 6.1 for more information about protecting the back. Make sure friends and family who assist frequently read that chapter also.
- Tell your assistant where to stand.
- Indicate how to hold onto your wheelchair (e.g., "Please do not lift from the foot supports because it might break off. Hold the frame next to my knees instead").
- Give body mechanics suggestions (e.g., "Bend at your knees and keep your back straight").
- Always instruct your assistant to move on your count of three to coordinate the efforts of all parties.
- Remember to thank your assistant for the help.

Manually Rolling Your Wheelchair

It will be difficult or impossible to manually push your wheelchair with the motor engaged. Know how to explain the disengagement of the motors so an assistant can push you if necessary. Be sure you know where the motors are located and how to operate the motor disconnect system.

Describing Safe Body Mechanics to the Spotter or Assistant

Be sure to protect your spotter or assistant from injury by reminding her to watch her body position. Remind your spotter or assistant to:

- Bend at the knees, not at the waist.
- Use her legs for strength rather than the weaker muscles of the back or arms. This will help prevent back strain.
- Keep her knees bent, not locked straight.
- Never twist at the waist. Instead, she should keep her torso facing the same direction as her hips. This will help prevent back strain.
- Keep her back straight. Hunching over or rounding at the shoulders can cause back strain.
- Keep breathing. Sometimes people forget to breathe when they are involved in physical activity. When someone holds their breath, they are more likely to tense their muscles and when their muscles are tense, they are more prone to strain and injury.

When You Do Not Want or Need Assistance

Sometimes people will try to help even when you do not ask. This can be very frustrating.

- A simple "Thanks, but I would like to do this by myself" or "Thank you, but it is actually easier for me to do this without assistance" can be effective.
- "Please don't grab my wheelchair" or a similar instruction is sometimes necessary for the more aggressive helper.

Experiencing New Environments

It is important to have assistance available when you try things for the first time (e.g., your first time using a crosswalk with curb ramps). Having a companion along to both spot and assist makes it safer to experiment with new or different skills.

The goal is to develop full independence. This does not necessarily mean that you will be able to perform all skills independently. Rather, it means that you are able to understand when and where you may need assistance, how to ask for it, and how to instruct others to assist safely.

Section 2.2

Learning Your Limits

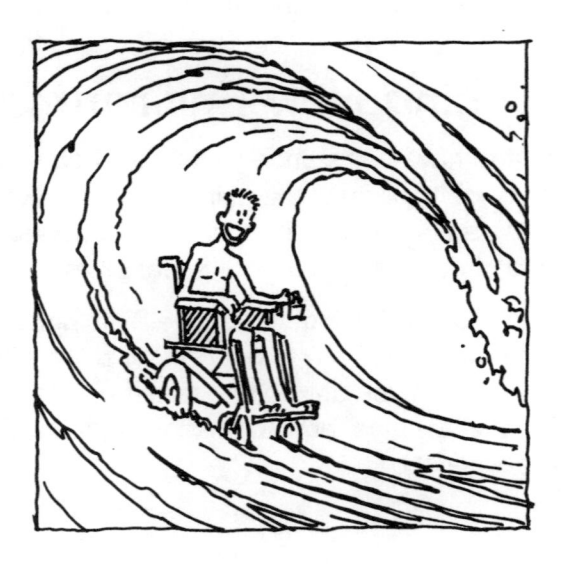

Riding at different speeds, going up and down hills, over different surfaces and past obstacles affects your stability. Depending on the terrain and your speed, you might have difficulty keeping your balance or your hand on the joystick. It is important to know your limits. To learn what you can do, you have to experience a variety of situations. Each time you try something new, it is best to have another person stand by to help you regain your balance and prevent you from falling. That person is referred to as a spotter throughout this book.

Techniques for Keeping Your Weight Back

Hitting an obstacle, coming to an abrupt stop or driving down a ramp, curb ramp or hill can all cause you to fall forward. Shifting your weight back in your wheelchair might help you keep your balance.

In order to counteract falling forward, it is important to stay as far back in your wheelchair as possible. Although the wheelchair's back support will prevent you from leaning back very far, leaning even your head and shoulders back will help keep you in your wheelchair. If you tend to lose your balance or fall forward, the following suggestions might be useful to you.

Hook your arm behind you

Hooking will help keep your body "locked against the back of your wheelchair." You will need sufficient arm movement and strength to position your arm and hold the push handle in the crook of your elbow. You may find that hooking your non-driving arm around the push handle will provide added stability while driving over obstacles or down ramps.

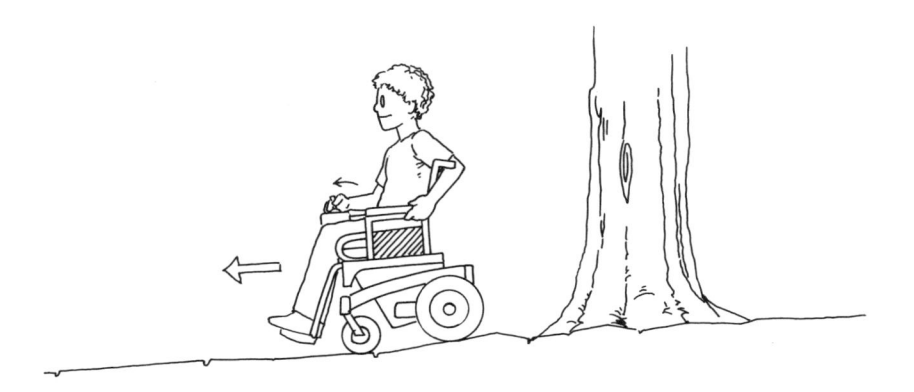

Hooking your arm can help you keep your balance when you ride downhill or over rough ground in your powered wheelchair.

Since hooking requires you to twist and lean, using this technique over many years can lead to back pain, pressure ulcers on your buttocks, and skeletal deformation. Hooking also occupies an arm that might be better used for other activities. If you find you need to hook often to feel safe while driving, you may want to obtain additional postural supports to minimize usage of this technique. Extended lateral supports or a chest support might be of great benefit.

Use of additional straps

A lap belt will help hold your buttocks back and keep you from sliding forward in your seat. Sliding forward in your seat could allow you to get dumped out on the ground. A lap belt can be positioned at different angles; however, a strap that crosses your thighs at an angle between 60 and 90 degrees will work the best.

A chest strap can help hold your upper body in place, preventing you from falling forward. Different styles are available depending on your needs and preferences. An alternative to the traditional chest strap is an across-the-shoulder automotive style belt or backpack style straps that come down across each shoulder.

Chest straps should be used with great care, because if you slide down (or forward) in your wheelchair, a chest strap can get caught around your throat and choke you. Chest straps of any type should only be used with a properly functioning lap belt.

> ### WARNING!
> Lap belts mounted at angles less than 60 degrees have the potential of pivoting up, and can allow the hips to slide underneath and forward on the wheelchair seat. For people using a chest support of some type, sliding down in the wheelchair can create a strangulation hazard. People have also slid down in their wheelchairs such that the lap belt created a strangulation hazard.

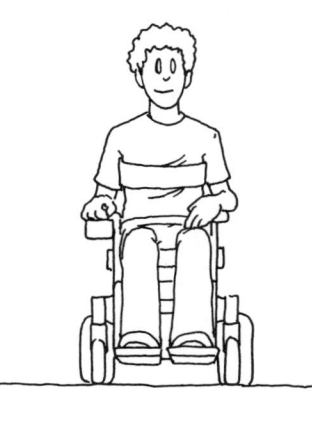

A chest strap in combination with a lap belt can help you maintain your sitting balance. Try several chest support styles to see what works best for you.

Power recline back support

If your wheelchair is equipped with power recline, you can adjust the back support rearward to prevent you from losing forward stability. The next section discusses this type of seating system in more detail.

Chapter Two: General Skills

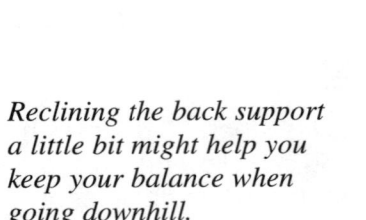

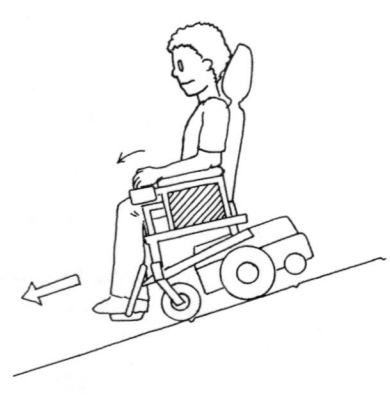

Reclining the back support a little bit might help you keep your balance when going downhill.

CAUTION

Never recline your back support when traveling uphill. This could lead to rearward instability when driving uphill, through a curb ramp or other uphill sloped situation.

Power tilt-in-space seating system

In a power tilt-in-space seating system the entire seating system tilts back, not just the back support. This type of seating system is discussed in more detail in the next section.

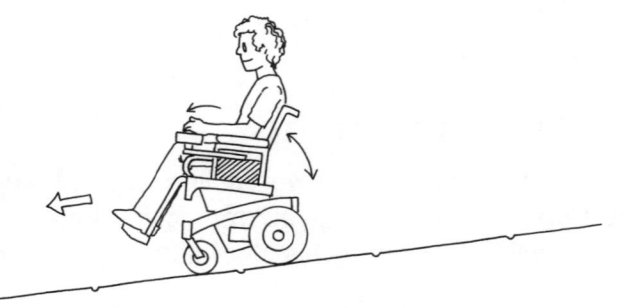

A power tilt-in-space feature can also help you keep your balance when going downhill.

CAUTION

Never use the power tilt feature when traveling uphill. This could lead to rearward instability when driving uphill, through a curb ramp or other uphill sloped situation.

Techniques for Keeping Your Weight Forward

When traveling uphill, you may need to keep your weight forward to prevent your wheelchair from tipping backward.

- Lean forward with your head and shoulders when driving over obstacles and when driving up hills and ramps.
- If you use a chest strap, it may be easier to lean forward against the strap with it slightly loosened.

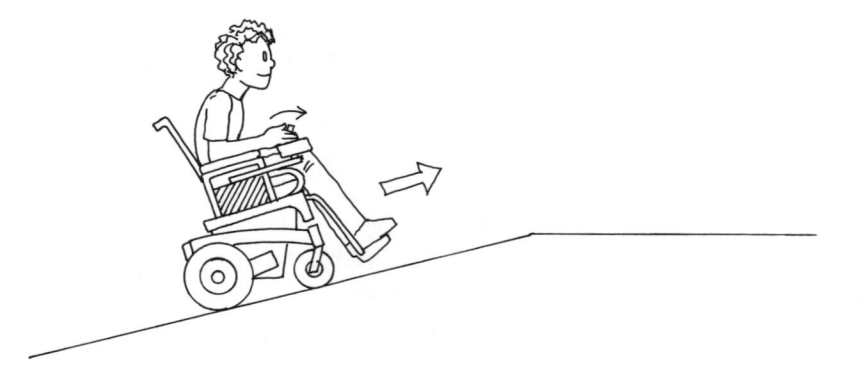

When traveling up a steep hill, you may need to keep your weight forward to prevent your wheelchair from tipping backward.

When You are Learning Your Limits

- First learn your balance point when sitting in your powered wheelchair. With a spotter's assistance, find out how steep a ramp (forward, rearward and sideways) you can handle before you start to lose your balance.
- Try different postural supports to see which will help you maintain your upper body balance.
- Learn to recognize environments that are beyond your ability to maintain your postural stability. Learn how to recognize ramps that are too steep for you to manage.
- Have a spotter stand by to help you regain your balance and prevent you from falling.

Chapter Two: General Skills

Section 2.3

Relieving Pressure

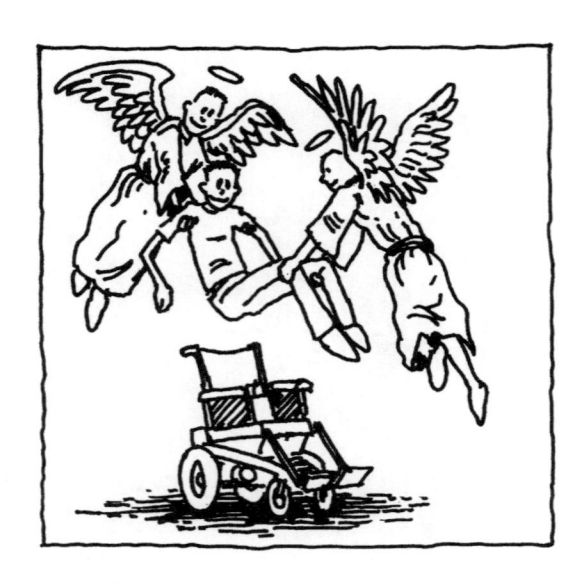

A weight shift lessens the pressure under your buttocks and thighs and helps blood flow to your legs and buttocks. **It is recommended that you perform a pressure relief weight shift at least every 10 to 20 minutes** to prevent pressure ulcers from developing. Weight shifts should last anywhere from 8 seconds to 1 minute. When choosing a method to do a weight shift make sure the pressure is relieved under both of your ischial bones (the bones you sit on).

If you are unable to perform any of the following weight shifting techniques, or if they are inadequate to prevent your skin from getting red after sitting, you should periodically get out of your wheelchair to lie on your side or stomach.

Forward Weight Shift

Resting on your thighs

- Lean your chest toward your knees, reaching down the frame of the chair.
- If you want to raise your buttocks higher, fold or remove your foot supports and position your feet on the floor. Try this first with a spotter to be certain you do not fall forward out of the wheelchair.
- Alternatively, you can lean forward with your elbows on your knees or on the arm supports of your wheelchair.

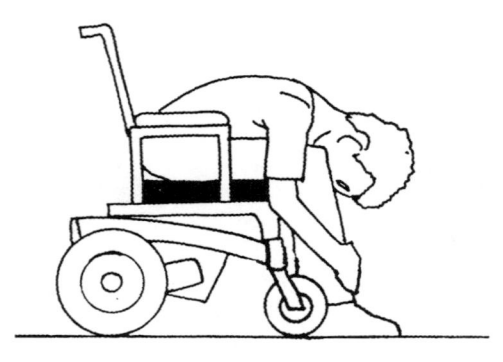

Leaning forward onto your thighs helps relieve sitting pressures.

Section 2.3: Relieving Pressure

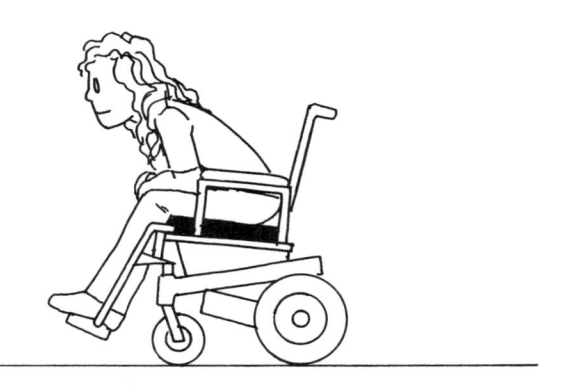

You can also lean on your knees to do a pressure relief weight shift.

Resting on a table

- Place a pillow on a desk or table.
- Lean forward and rest on the pillow.
- Use the desk or table to push yourself up when finished.
- Be sure to have a spotter check that you have completely unweighted your buttocks. Your spotter's hand should be able to feel little pressure between your buttocks and the cushion.

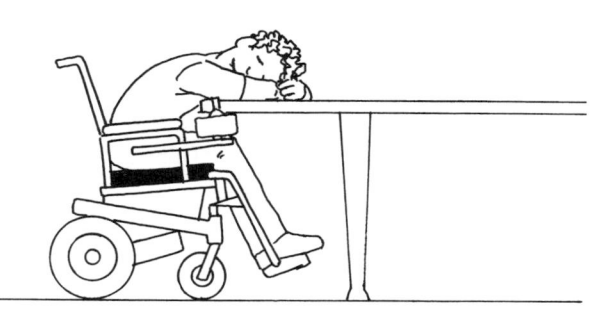

Leaning forward on a table is another way to unweight your buttocks during a pressure relief.

Leaning from the push handles

- Hook one or both of your arms around the push handles behind you.
- Lean forward.

Using weight shift loops

If you do not have good triceps strength, weight shift loops can help you perform a forward weight shift. Weight shift loops are looped straps attached to the back of a chair that help those without triceps strength perform a forward weight shift.

- Put your hands in the looped portion of your lifting straps or weight shift loops and lean forward.
- Pull yourself up with the weight shift loops when ready to sit upright again.

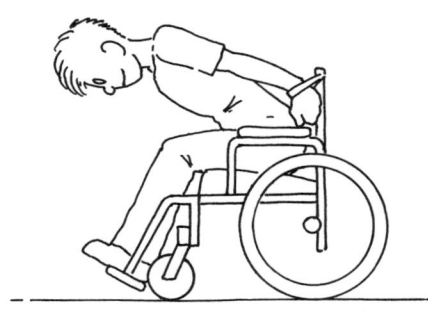

Weight shift loops might help you perform a forward pressure relief if your triceps are weak.

Side-to-Side Weight Shift

Side-to-side weight shifts relieve pressure on one buttock at a time. Make sure you lean to each side so both sides of your buttocks get unweighted.

- Pull up parallel to a desk, counter, wall or bed, and place the forearm closest to the object on its surface. Lean on the supported forearm.

- With your other hand, grasp the far arm support and push up and toward the desk. Be sure your buttocks clear the seat.
- Turn around and do this maneuver on the other side.

Alternatively, you can:
- Place both hands or elbows on the arm support.
- Lean to one side, alternately lifting each buttock until it clears the seat.
- Have a spotter check to see if you have leaned far enough to create space under your buttocks.

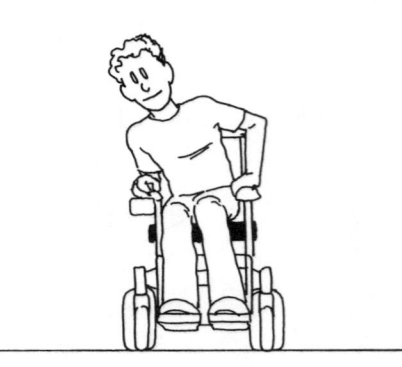

Lean to one side to unweight the other side.

Push Up Weight Shift

Triceps strength is necessary to perform this type of weight shift.
- Place your hands on the arm supports, wheels or other part of the wheelchair.
- Push down through your hands until your arms are straight and your buttocks have lifted off the seat.

Weight Shift Through Powered Seating

Some people are unable to perform any of the above weight shifts. Powered wheelchairs are now available with power recline and tilt features that are controlled by a switch near your joystick. The switches can often be repositioned to a different location depending on your needs.

Power recline back support

This type of seating has a mechanism that will recline the back support and open the seat-to-back angle.

- Some wheelchairs have leg supports that elevate independently of the back support. Some wheelchairs with power recline have leg supports that are linked to the back support, allowing you to raise your legs as you recline your back.
- As you recline, your position may change in relation to your lateral supports, head support and other postural supports. This might cause discomfort and improper support.
- If the seating system has a "zero sheer" back support that moves with your back as you recline, your postural supports should not move relative to your body when you recline the back support.

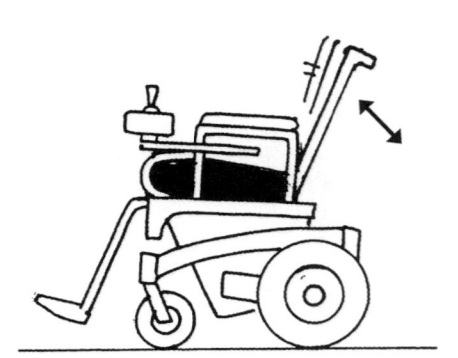

The back support of some wheelchairs can be reclined back.

Power tilt-in-space seating system

In a tilt-in-space seating system, the back support and seat of the wheelchair tip forward or backward together, changing the orientation of the entire seating system to the wheelbase. This moves your entire body into a tilted position without changing the angle of your hip and knee joints. If you use power tilt for pressure relief weight shifts, you will need to tilt all the way back to shift the weight off your buttocks to allow the blood to properly circulate. Sometimes tilt-in-space seating is preferred over reclining, because your body does not move in relation to your postural supports.

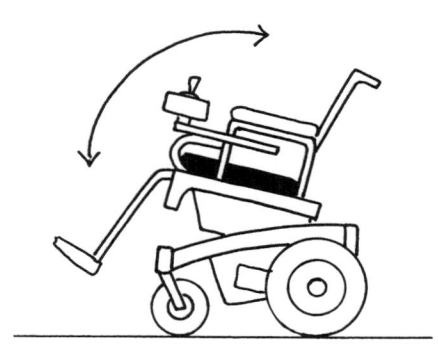

With a tilt-in-space wheelchair, the back reclines and the seat tips up together.

Recline and tilt seating

A combination of power recline and power tilt, while more complex, might make weight shifts and other movements easier. A combination allows you to move the back support of the wheelchair forward and back and change the angle of the seat, either at the same time or independently of one another.

Section 2.4

Reaching, Bending and Lifting

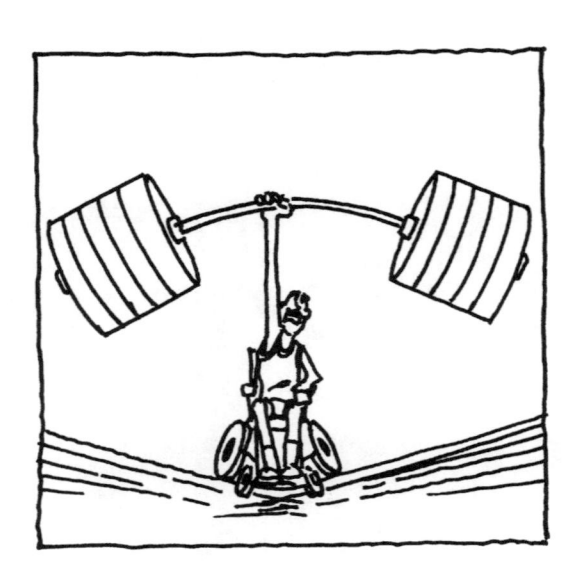

Aside from helping you get where you want to go, your trusty wheelchair provides a platform for you to do things once you arrive at your destination. "Doing things" often involves reaching and moving objects. Bending, reaching and lifting may not be easy. How you perform these skills depends largely on what you are trying to do. With practice, you will be able to develop easier or alternate ways to reach for or lift different objects. Practice reaching for and lifting objects of different sizes and weights.

Avoid reaching across your body, especially when reaching for something you would not want to have fall in your lap, such as hot coffee or a sharp knife. Twisting and lifting at the same time increases the risk of straining your back, so be careful when lifting from the side. Never try to reach for or lift objects that might exceed your capabilities. Ask for help when lifting heavy or awkward objects. Some people use trained service dogs to pick up and retrieve objects.

If you want to get a light object off a high store shelf, ask for assistance. If no one is available to help, use another product in the store, such as a cereal box, to knock the item off the shelf. Never knock heavy or breakable objects off a shelf.

Before you reach, put your casters in a trailing position pointed toward the direction of the reach. This will lengthen your wheelbase and improve your stability (see Section 2.5 for more information about caster trail).

Reaching Sideways

If possible, pull up next to, rather than in front of, an object and reach to the side. You may have more trunk stability than if you try to reach forward or backward.

Objects on a counter or at counter height

- Pull up next to the counter.
- Reach to the side for the object.
- If you need to, hold onto the opposite arm support or push handle to help stabilize yourself.

Section 2.4: Reaching, Bending and Lifting

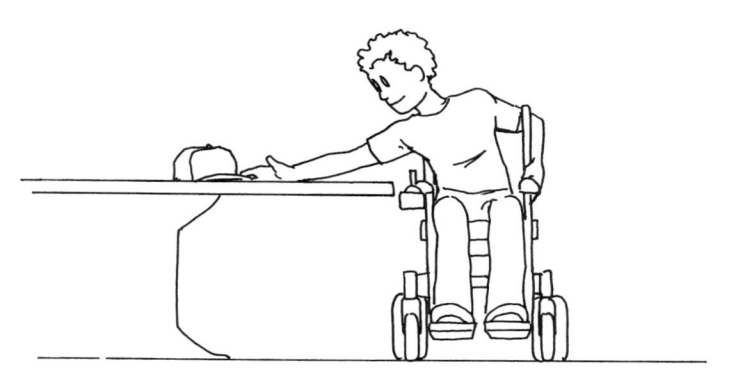

Holding onto the arm supports affords more stability when reaching sideways.

Objects on the ground or on a low shelf

- Pull up so the object is to the side of your wheelchair.
- Hook your arm or wrist around the push handle or grab the arm supports on the side of the wheelchair opposite the object.
- Lean down to pick up the object with your free arm.
- When you have grasped the object, pull yourself up with your other arm around the push handle or the arm support of the wheelchair.

How a spotter can help

- Stand to the side of the wheelchair opposite the object the wheelchair rider is lifting.
- Be ready to keep the wheelchair rider from falling forward out of the wheelchair.
- Be ready to assist the wheelchair rider back upright if needed.

Reaching Forward

The ability to reach forward is useful to tie your shoes, pick up objects from the floor or to empty a leg bag. You can use your foot supports, feet and/or knees to help lift the object into your lap.

Avoid reaching for objects with your weaker hand. Instead, turn around and use your stronger hand to grasp and lift.

Basic forward reach

- Lean forward with one forearm laid across your knees or firmly grab the wheelchair frame in front of the seat for support, then reach forward with the other hand.
- Lift the object onto your feet or foot supports.
- Push your free forearm against your knees or push down on the wheelchair frame with a hand to raise yourself up, pulling the object into your lap at the same time.

Braced forward reach

- Bend forward, resting your chest on your knees. Reach forward with one hand and lift the object onto your feet or foot supports.
- Hook the other arm or wrist around the push handle or back of the wheelchair and pull yourself up.
- Leaning forward slightly, grab the object and lift it onto your lap.

Diagonal forward reach

- Hook an arm or wrist around the back of your wheelchair.
- Bend forward and rest your upper body on your knee, bracing yourself with the arm or wrist hooked around the push handle or wheelchair back.
- Reach forward with your free hand and lift the object onto your feet or directly into your lap.
- Pull yourself upright using the arm hooked around the push handle or back of your wheelchair.

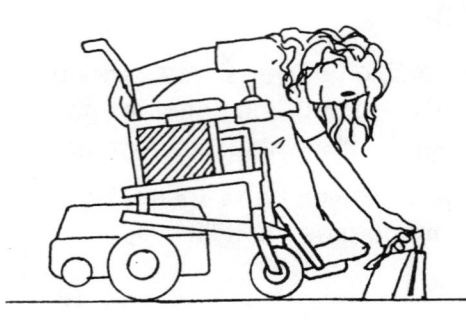

Use one back post or push handle to brace yourself when reaching forward.

How a spotter can help

- Be sure the casters are in a rearward trailing position pointed toward the object the wheelchair rider is trying to reach.
- Stand to the side of the wheelchair opposite the object the wheelchair rider is picking up.
- Be ready to keep the rider from falling out of the wheelchair.

Helpful Hints

There are many adaptive devices available to help you reach for objects, such as:

- a cane
- a dressing stick
- a reacher
- a hanger
- a button hook device
- double-sided tape on a ruler
- a magnet on a stick
- tongs (barbecue and scissors types)

Section 2.5

Main Wheel and Caster Management

Section 2.5: Main Wheel and Caster Management

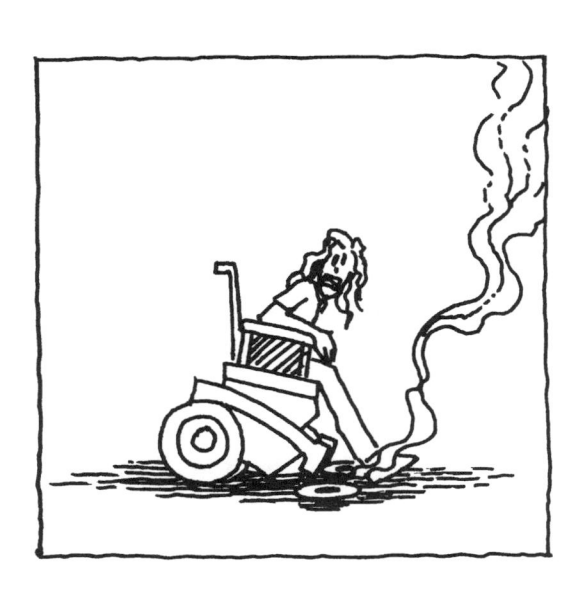

The position, size, composition, and condition of the main wheels and casters affect the performance and stability of a wheelchair. Powered wheelchairs usually do not have tire size and wheel positioning options.

Wheel Position

Wheel position affects wheelchair stability. A wheelchair with a wide or long wheelbase will be more stable than one with a narrow or short wheelbase. Many manufacturers do not provide for or recommend main wheel adjustments because such adjustments might impair the overall performance and stability of the chair.

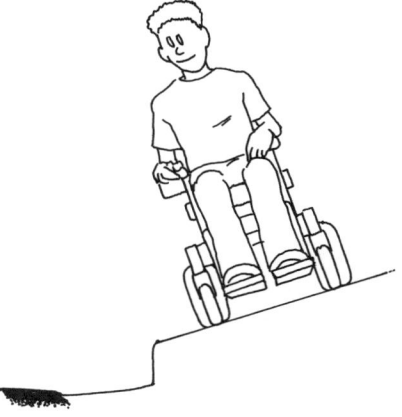

A wide wheelbase is more stable than a narrow one.

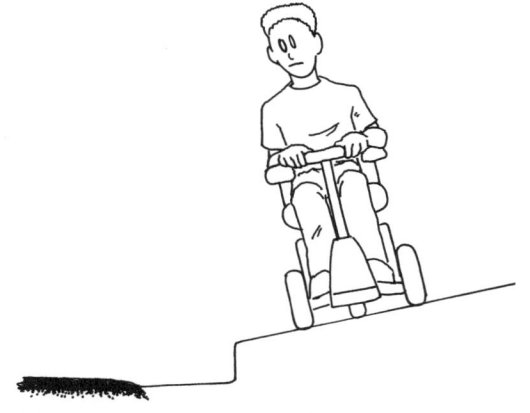

Many scooters that are designed for indoor mobility have wheelbase widths that are on the narrow side.

41

Chapter Two: General Skills

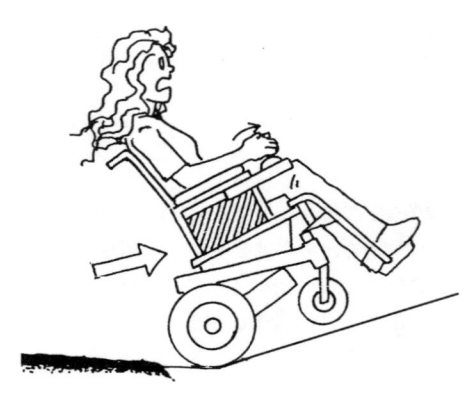

The bottom of a curb ramp and other similar grade transitions can cause a powered wheelchair with a short wheelbase to tip backward.

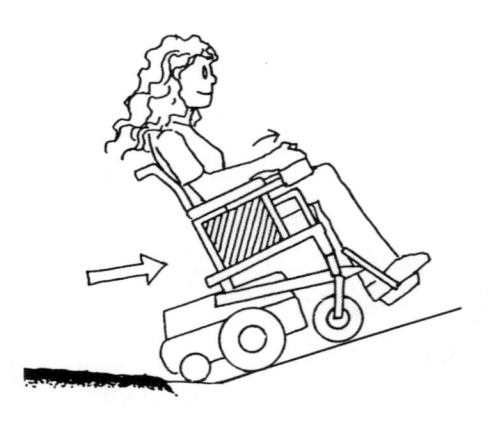

Many mid-wheel drive powered chairs have spring-loaded anti-tippers that create an effectively longer wheelbase and limit the amount of tipping in the rearward direction.

Wheel Size

The footprint of the wheels influences the ride and ability to traverse obstacles.

- The footprint is the amount of the wheel's tire that comes in contact with the ground at any given point.
- Larger wheels (diameter and width) usually have larger footprints; smaller wheels usually have smaller footprints.
- Wheels with large footprints help you drive over rough terrain and obstacles, but can reduce your range on smooth surfaces because there is more friction. Range is equivalent to mileage in a car, or how far you will be able to travel on a fully charged battery.

Composition

The composition of the wheel can affect its footprint. Soft main wheels and casters, like those filled (or partially filled) with air, flatten and create larger footprints. Pneumatic tires are better suited to use on rough terrain and over obstacles but carry the risk of going flat. Hard tires, like those made of solid rubber or those with flat-free inserts, create smaller footprints and are better suited to driving on smooth, hard surfaces. It is important to determine what kinds of surfaces you will be traveling on, as well as the availability of replacement parts when you choose a particular type of wheelchair.

Condition

As your tires wear out, the wheelchair's performance will change. Just as with car tires, the tread is meant to give you more traction and help you traverse obstacles. As the tread wears smooth, you are more likely to slip.

If you have pneumatic (air-filled) tires, it is important to keep them filled. When the tires are under-inflated, your wheelchair will act sluggish and lose range. If one tire is softer than the other, the chair will tend to veer in the direction of the softer tire. Improperly inflated tires may impair your side-to-side balance as well.

If you have solid tires, be aware that they dry out over time, and cracks and divots can form as a result of driving over obstacles. Tires should be replaced when the ride of your wheelchair becomes uncomfortable or undesirable in any way.

… Section 2.5: Main Wheel and Caster Management

Caster Management and Caster Trail

The small wheels that swivel on your wheelchair are casters. Each caster is attached to the wheelchair frame by a caster fork.

- Caster forks have a bend in them so that as you travel, the casters trail along rather than being pushed.
- When you drive backward in a wheelchair with front casters, the casters will trail toward the front of the chair. This is called the rearward trailing position.
- When you drive forward, the casters trail toward the rear of the chair and are in the forward trailing position.

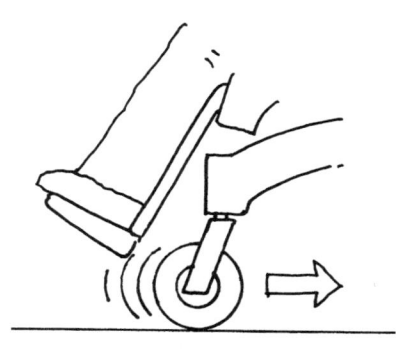

This is the rearward trailing position of the casters, which occurs when the chair is driven backwards.

This is the forward trailing position of the casters, which occurs when the chair is driven forwards.

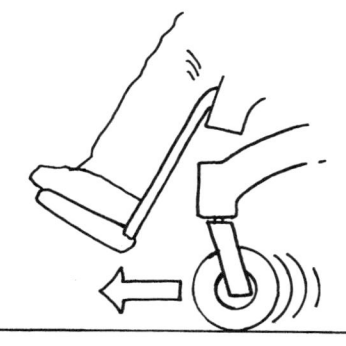

Pay attention to the position of your casters when you are traveling over obstacles and through cluttered environments. If the casters turn sideways they could get caught in crevices, stop your wheelchair abruptly and pitch you forward.

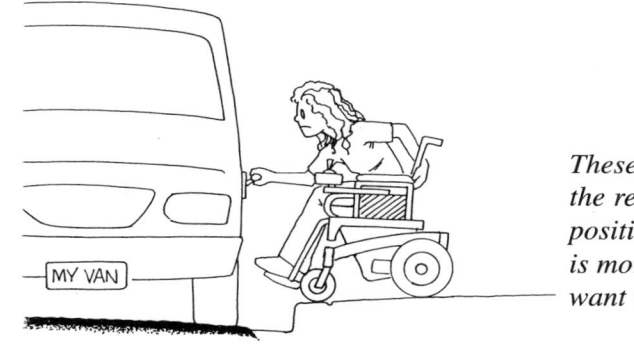

These casters are in the rearward trailing position. This position is more stable when you want to reach forward.

Exercises

Practice caster management by moving the joystick to change your caster position. If you can, lean over to watch the caster position change as you maneuver. If you cannot lean in your wheelchair, perform these exercises in front of a mirror so you can see your casters.

- Drive forward to face both casters in the forward trailing position.
- Move the casters into a rearward trailing position by driving in reverse for a short distance.
- Move your joystick to make full clockwise and counterclockwise rotations of the casters.
- If you drive your wheelchair forward and then stop, the casters will be in the forward trailing position. Now if you back up slowly you will notice that the front end of the wheelchair moves slightly left or right as the casters spin around. If you don't plan for this movement and the casters swivel the wrong

Chapter Two: General Skills

way in a tight environment, you can actually get stuck against a wall. Similarly, if you back into an elevator, the casters will be in the rearward trailing position. When you drive forward, the casters will swivel around and the front end of your chair will move slightly to the side as it moves forward. By moving forward a bit right after getting in, your casters will swivel into the forward trailing position and you will be ready to drive back out. Doing this before the elevator fills up with people will prevent your wheelchair casters from spinning around and hitting the toes of your fellow elevator passengers.

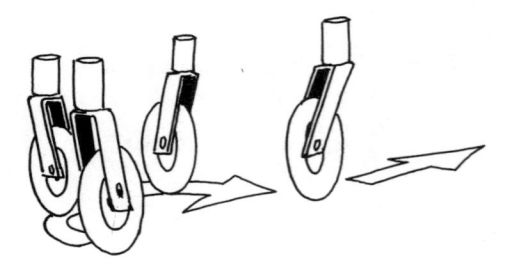

Spinning your casters in a desired direction can take practice.

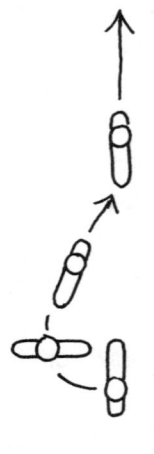

Practice moving your wheelchair so your casters spin in clockwise and counterclockwise directions.

Type of Caster

The manufacturer may offer a variety of caster types.

- The diameter generally varies from 8 to 12 inches.
- The width generally varies from 2 to 4 inches.
- In general, a larger, wider caster will decrease the maneuverability of the wheelchair in indoor environments but will improve outdoor maneuverability and obstacle-climbing ability.
- Pneumatic casters add an air cushion to the ride, increasing rider comfort. However, pneumatic casters require additional maintenance to keep them properly inflated and to fix flats.

Caster Flutter

The casters may vibrate back and forth, or flutter, when you travel at higher speeds. Caster flutter can cause rapid deceleration of the wheelchair on one side, resulting in decreased directional control. This problem can be corrected. The caster housing may be bent or out of adjustment. Some wheelchairs have an adjustment for the caster stem angle or the bearing to eliminate or reduce this problem. Slowing down will temporarily eliminate the problem. Special bushings are available for some wheelchairs with this problem.

Another method to reduce flutter is to increase the caster trail by using a different set of caster forks and/or complete caster assemblies.

CHAPTER 3

In this Chapter

3.1	Smooth Surfaces	47
3.2	Thresholds and Obstacles	48
3.3	Doorways and Tight Environments	53
3.4	Rough Terrain	63
3.5	Ramps	66
3.6	Cross Slopes	71
3.7	Curbs and Steps	74
3.8	Elevators and Platform Lifts	80
3.9	Tracks and Grates	85

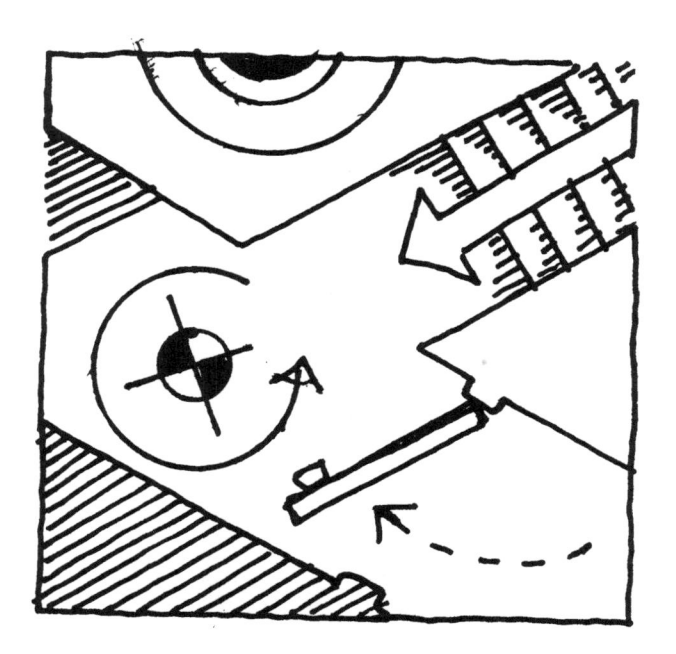

Navigation Skills

As just about everyone knows, the world isn't flat. Nor is it uniformly smooth, level, firm, stable, and slip resistant. There are still curbs to climb, doors to contend with and lawns to cross. Your wheelchair can help you access all of these types of terrain, sometimes independently and other times with assistance.

Before practicing the maneuvers in this section, read the warnings on page xi to learn about the risks involved in performing powered wheelchair maneuvers. Many of the skills in this section require significant wheelchair experience and good joystick control skills. Most people have fallen at some point while performing these maneuvers. For some wheelchair riders, falling could result in severe injury or death.

Chapter Three: Navigational Skills

> **WARNING!**
> Removing or repositioning your anti-tippers could allow your powered wheelchair to tip over backwards. This could result in injury or death. Always use the anti-tippers positioned as they were supplied by the manufacturer. Removing the anti-tippers should be done with extreme caution, and only after you have a clear understanding of the potential consequences and you have received proper training in the use of your wheelchair without the anti-tippers.

A note about anti-tippers: Most manufacturers send their powered wheelchairs out with some type of anti-tip device. Traditional anti-tippers are small wheels, 1 or 2 inches in diameter, and may be removable with or without tools. They may have to be repositioned or removed to have complete and independent mobility outside. Anti-tippers can get caught going through height transitions and small curbs, causing you to get "hung-up." Some anti-tippers can be repositioned to accomplish a specific maneuver, or removed and then reinstalled. While this may not be very practical, it is possible. Even when the anti-tippers are in place, they may not prevent a wheelchair from completely tipping over to the rear. If the wheelchair is on a slope steep enough to start tipping, you are in a situation that exceeds the design limits of the chair. Extreme caution should be used when operating your wheelchair on slopes approaching the design limits of your wheelchair. Some wheelchairs have large spring-loaded anti-tippers, which are designed to be driven on in certain situations.

You will note that many of the illustrations in this book show wheelchairs without anti-tip devices in place. The book has been illustrated this way because the majority of powered wheelchair users do not use anti-tippers.

Section 3.1

Smooth Surfaces

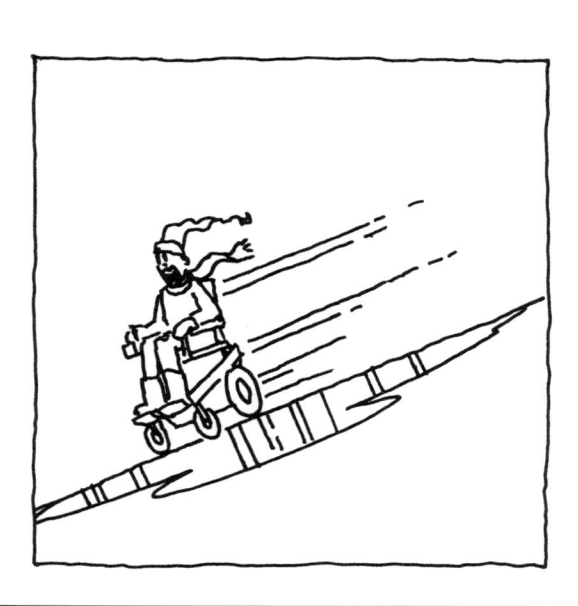

When you are driving a powered wheelchair, the surface over which you roll affects how your wheelchair will perform. Surfaces that allow optimal performance are smooth, level, firm, stable, and slip resistant. You will usually find this type of surface indoors, such as in public buildings like schools, offices and shopping malls. These surfaces are often made from hard wood, vinyl flooring or concrete. If you notice your chair performing awkwardly, such as pulling to one side while riding on a smooth, level surface, it is probably due to a problem with the wheelchair. In this instance, it might be a low tire or a motor malfunction on one side of the chair.

Crossing Smooth Surfaces

If the surface is firm, stable and slip resistant, crossing it is merely a matter of proper wheelchair driving technique (see Section 1.5 for more information about basic joystick operation). Still, watch out for:

- Changes in surface type, such as from wood to carpet
- Hazards such as push-pin tacks, glass or other sharp objects
- Objects that could get crushed, such as shoes or children's toys
- Low tire pressure in one wheel which can cause you to have difficulty maintaining directional control

Chapter Three: Navigational Skills

Section 3.2

Thresholds and Obstacles

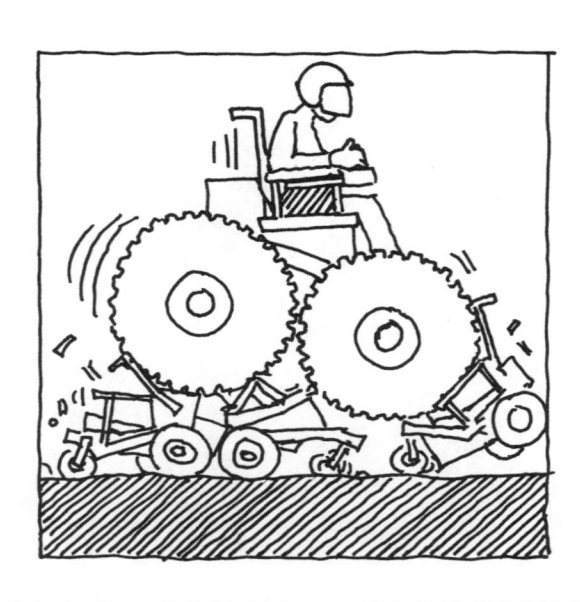

Before learning how to cross thresholds and negotiate obstacles, you should be able to drive forward, backward and turn while managing the orientation of the casters (see Section 2.5 on caster management for more details on this often overlooked issue). Minimal trunk control is needed to cross low thresholds and obstacles. As the obstacle height increases, trunk control and balance become more important.

In any type of obstacle negotiation, a shoulder or chest strap can help you maintain your upper body balance. If you do not have a chest strap, ask your spotter or assistant to be prepared to catch your upper body if you lose your balance.

Foot Support Clearance

The positioning of your foot supports is very important. A foot support in a low position can catch on thresholds, curb ramps and other obstacles.

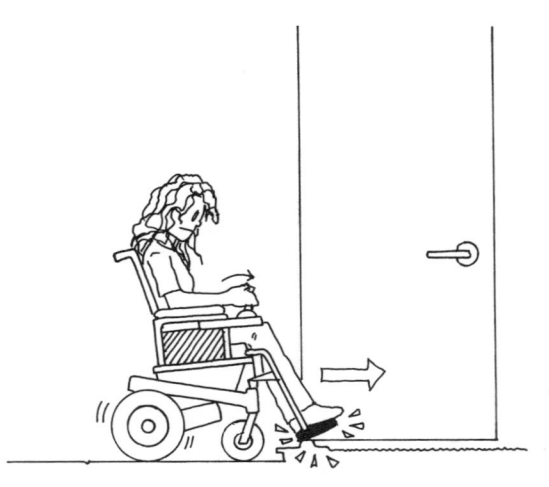

Your foot supports might get caught on a threshold or other obstacle if there is not enough foot support clearance.

When driving through a slope transition at the base of a curb ramp, the foot supports of any wheelchair will be closer to the ground. When the foot supports contact a solid object, the wheelchair can come to an abrupt stop. You can be thrown forward completely out of the wheelchair if a lap belt is not worn. Worse yet, the entire wheelchair could tip in the forward direction, landing on top of you. For this reason, it is common to have the foot supports at least 2 inches off the ground.

If this causes your thighs to be unsupported on your cushion, raise your seat or use a thicker seat cushion. Consider using foot supports with high density plastic skid plates or wheels. These features are designed to deflect the footrests in the forward direction upon contact with the ground to prevent abrupt stops. These will help prevent you from getting stuck on a curb ramp or other obstacle.

Crossing a Door Threshold or Obstacle

A threshold is the raised bump in a doorway that prevents water and air drafts from leaking into a room. Usually made of wood or metal, thresholds vary in height and can be barriers to some powered wheelchairs. Modified rear-wheel drive wheelchairs with large front casters can climb over thresholds and obstacles more easily than chairs with smaller casters, which may catch on objects in the path of travel. Door thresholds and any obstacles less than ½ inch in height usually do not present difficulties for powered wheelchairs. Your ability to drive over a threshold or obstacle of greater heights will depend on the wheelchair and the type of obstacle.

Take safety precautions when learning to cross thresholds and obstacles. If you have poor trunk balance, try using a chest strap for more trunk support. Always have a spotter nearby to catch your upper body in case you start losing your balance while practicing.

Moving over a threshold or obstacle essentially requires two crossings: one to move the front wheels over, and the other to bring the rear wheels over. If the surface on the other side of the obstacle is higher than the one you are starting from, it will generally be more comfortable to go in the forward direction. If the surface on the other side of the obstacle is lower than the one you are starting from, it may be more comfortable to cross the obstacle backward, unless you are comfortable tipping forward. For wheelchairs with the drive wheels in the rear, sometimes riding backward over obstacles is easier and more effective. This is especially true if the surface on the other side of the obstacle is lower than the one you are starting from.

Quite often, additional power needs to be applied to the chair to cross a threshold or obstacle. When the casters finally cross the obstacle, the chair may lunge forward. Chairs with the drive wheels in the front are better at climbing over small obstacles, where the casters are pulled over behind the main drive wheels.

Crossing a threshold or obstacle independently

Once you learn your limits and become familiar with driving your powered wheelchair, you will learn which obstacles to avoid or go around and which ones to go over. You can cross thresholds and obstacles by driving in either the forward or reverse direction. Depending on the wheel configuration of your wheelchair and the height of the obstacle, it may be easier to cross the obstacle first with the drive wheels and with the casters trailing over last. This could mean that for some situations the preferred direction of travel would be backward. Mid-wheel drive wheelchairs generally climb obstacles best in the forward direction with the front casters crossing the obstacle first. Be careful not to get stuck with your casters on one side of the threshold or obstacle and the rear wheels on the other. A railroad track is an example of this potential situation (see Section 3.9).

Here are some good tips for crossing a threshold or obstacle independently.

- Check for sufficient foot support clearance.
- Check for anti-tipper clearance. It may be necessary to remove or reposition the anti-tippers to prevent you from getting caught on a threshold.
- Decide if you want to cross the threshold or obstacle driving forward or backward.

- Approach and contact the threshold as perpendicular as possible so both casters cross at the same time, resulting in a smoother, less bumpy transition than driving over one wheel at a time in a diagonal direction.
- Move the joystick in the direction needed to drive over the threshold or obstacle.
- Drive at a slow speed and gradually increase your speed after the front wheels contact and climb the obstacle.
- Stopping with the front wheels against the obstacle and then applying forward power is another way to get the casters up and over an obstacle.
- Move forward slowly as the casters travel up and over the obstacle, and then apply additional power as the rear wheels cross the obstacle.

You may want to practice this technique with a spotter behind you until you learn what size obstacle you can cross without danger of tipping over to the rear.

How a spotter can help

If the wheelchair user can get the casters up onto the obstacle but cannot get the rear wheels up, you can assist in the following manner:

- Stand behind the wheelchair with one hand close to the push handles or the back posts and the other positioned over one of the rider's shoulders.
- Be ready to catch the rider at the shoulders if the rider loses balance in the forward direction.
- Place one foot in front of the other and use your body weight to push forward against the back of the wheelchair.
- Put your weight into the chair when the rider applies forward power to the wheelchair.

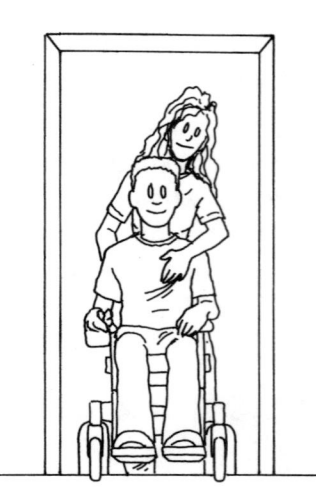

Stand behind the user with a hand over the shoulder, ready to catch the user if balance is lost.

Crossing a threshold or obstacle with assistance

If you feel uncomfortable crossing a threshold or obstacle and there is no alternative route, ask for help.

- Drive forward and check for foot support clearance. If your foot supports hit the threshold or obstacle first, have your assistant "tip" the wheelchair back far enough to clear the foot supports by pushing down on the back of the chair as you drive forward.
- If there is sufficient foot support clearance, drive the wheelchair forward until your front wheels rest against the threshold or obstacle.
- Have the assistant hold onto the chair from the back.
- Ask your assistant to push down and back on the push handles while you drive the wheelchair forward. This will help raise the casters high enough to "climb" the threshold or obstacle.

Section 3.2: Thresholds and Obstacles

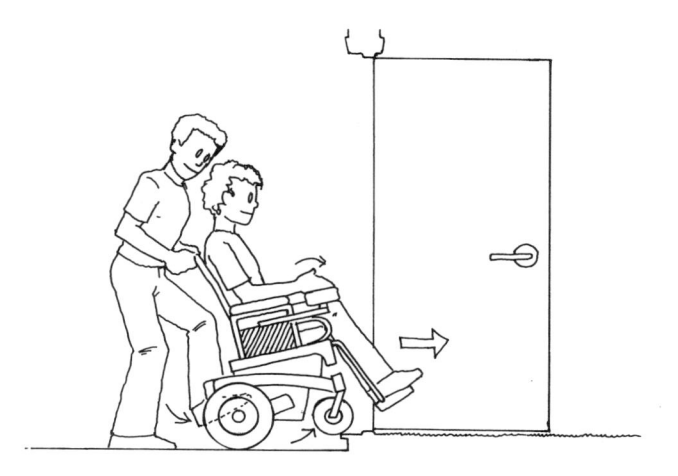

Pushing down and forward simultaneously on the push handles helps to lift the front casters so they can climb up an obstacle.

- After the casters are up on top of the obstacle, ask your assistant to push up and forward on the back of the chair while you apply forward power.
- Continue to drive forward until your rear wheels cross over the threshold or obstacle.

WARNING!

A high threshold can stop the wheelchair when the front casters contact the threshold. After supplying sufficient power, the casters can pop up over the obstacle. This can cause the wheelchair to tip back, so have a spotter behind you when attempting to climb over high thresholds.

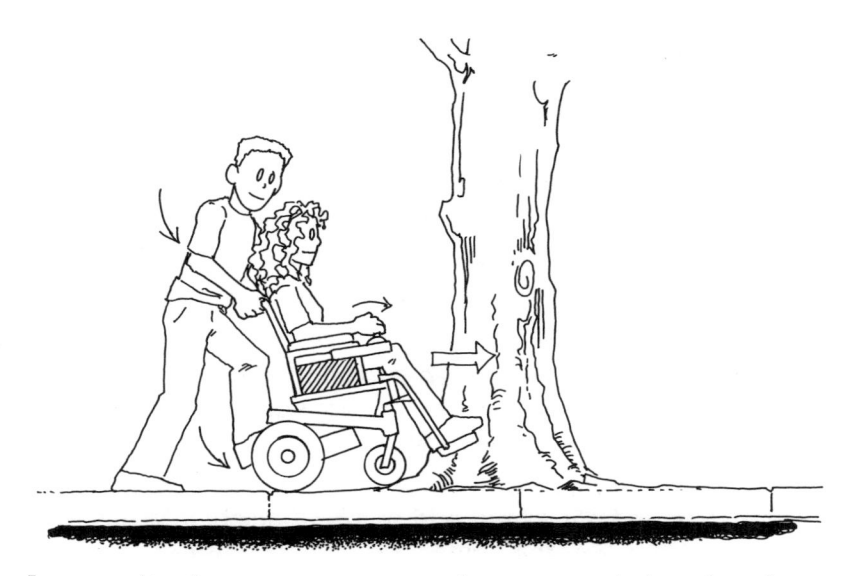

In some situations you may want assistance negotiating obstacles such as tree roots.

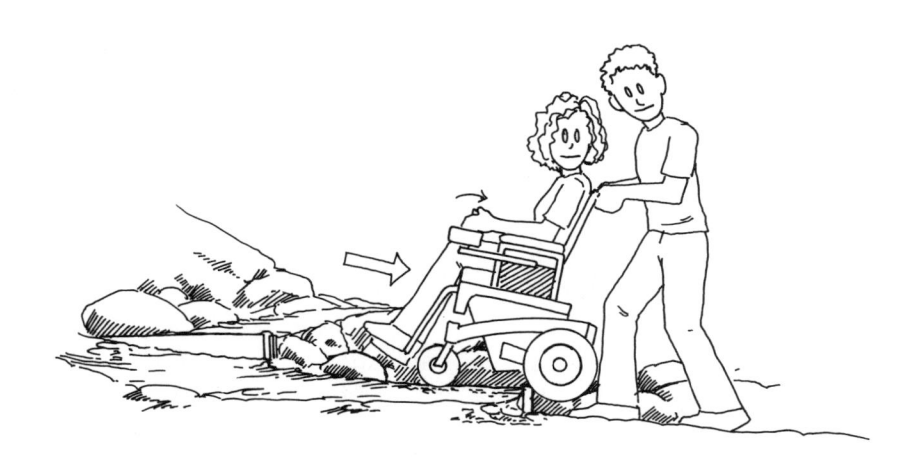

With drive wheels in the rear, sometimes maneuvering backward over obstacles is easier and more effective.

Crossing a threshold or obstacle with assistance – alternative method

Ask your assistant to:

- Stand to the side of the wheelchair.
- If two assistants are available, have the second assistant stand in back of the wheelchair and hold onto the push handles.
- Have your assistant at the side bend at the knees and grab the frame of the wheelchair near the front caster.
- Your assistant should be prepared to lift the front end of the wheelchair high enough to clear the foot supports over the obstacle as you slowly drive forward.
- On the count of three, slowly apply forward power as your assistant lifts up on the front end of the wheelchair to guide the front casters over the obstacle.
- Stop when the wheelchair has straddled the obstacle.
- Have your assistant move to the back of the wheelchair to help the rear wheels over the obstacle by pushing forward and up as you drive forward over the obstacle.

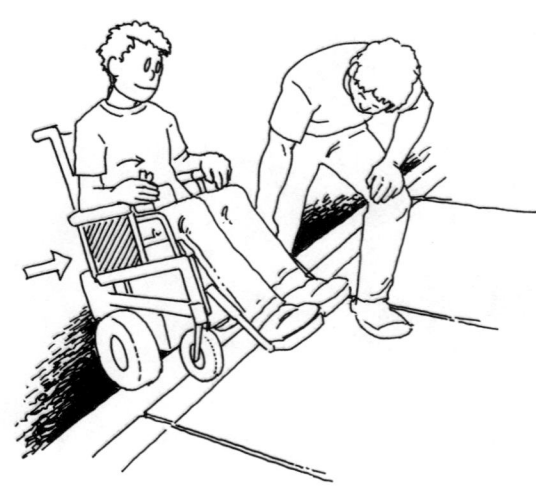

Sometimes you will need an assistant to lift the front of the wheelchair, as you slowly drive forward, to negotiate a curb, threshold or obstacle.

Section 3.3

Doorways and Tight Environments

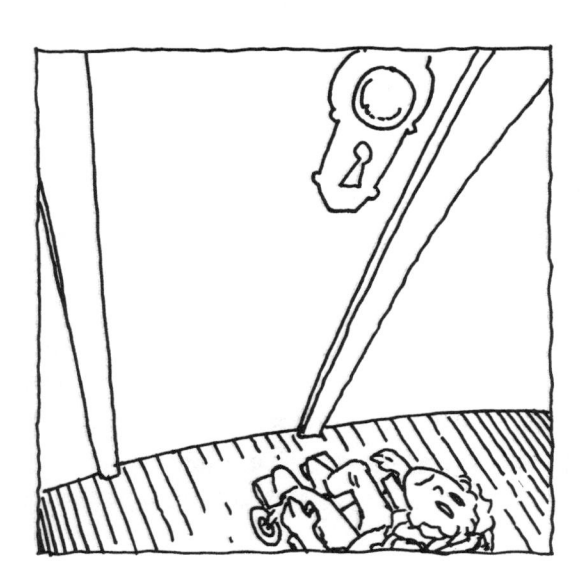

Doorways can pose significant challenges. Negotiating a doorway requires you to maneuver within a constricted space, to open a door and its latch, and travel up and over a threshold. The Americans with Disabilities Act (ADA) Accessibility Guidelines have set design standards that will allow most wheelchairs to use doorways. The ADA Accessibility Guidelines specify that doors must have a passageway at least 32 inches wide, should have a handle instead of a knob, and should be able to be opened with less than a 5 pound force. The ADA Accessibility Guidelines also state that the threshold should be no more than a half inch in height. If you regularly encounter a door that is difficult to open, speak to the building's management to see if the force used to open the door can be reduced. See Appendix A on the ADA for more information.

If a door knob or handle is difficult to operate, ask someone to open it for you. Levers are easier to use than round knobs. Some levers are essentially handle extensions that can be installed over existing knobs, while others will replace the latch as well. Door levers are usually available at hardware stores.

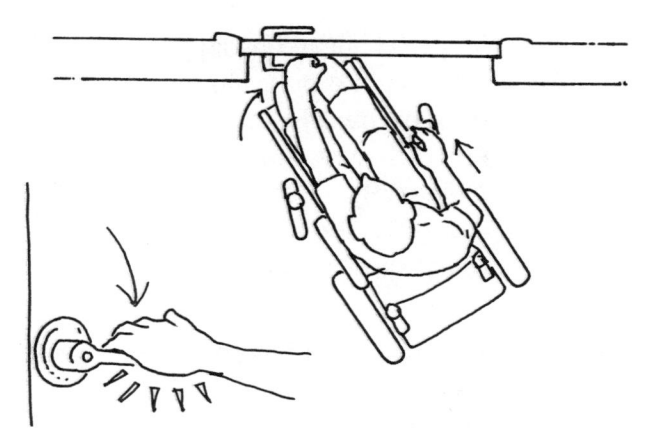

Levers are usually easier to manage than doorknobs.

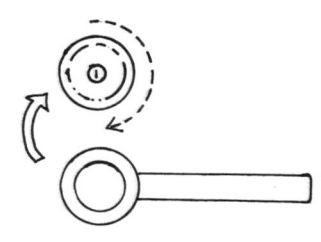

Round door knobs can be very difficult to grip if you have limited hand function. A lever can be placed over the knob, making it easier to turn.

Chapter Three: Navigational Skills

Before learning the skills in this section, you should be able to drive a wheelchair, reach for objects, and cross thresholds. Always have a spotter nearby when learning to open doors and move through tight environments.

How a spotter can help with all manual doors

When reaching forward for the door handle or crossing the threshold, the rider could lose trunk stability and fall forward. Catch the rider at the shoulder to prevent this from happening.

Stand to the side of the wheelchair and place a hand on or near the shoulder to keep the rider from falling forward. If falling forward is a problem for the wheelchair rider, a chest strap can be used.

Manual Swinging Doors

With a spotter nearby, practice opening, closing, and driving through doors in bathroom stalls, entryways and public buildings. If you think you will have difficulty leaning to reach a door handle, ask your spotter to stand to one side and be prepared to catch you at the trunk if you lose your balance (see Section 2.4 for more information about bending and reaching). Try to let the power of the wheelchair do most of the work. The motion of driving the wheelchair forward and backward can be used to pull and push the door.

Driving through a doorway usually involves crossing a raised threshold (see Section 3.2 for more information about crossing thresholds). Whether you are able to open certain doors depends on which side of the wheelchair your joystick drive control is on and how much function you have in the other arm.

Free-swinging doors

- Make sure the bottom of the door is not glass, which can shatter. Many doors have kick plates for this purpose.

- If the door swings and does not latch shut, approach the door at an angle from the direction of the hinges toward the side of the door that swings.
- Use your foot supports to push the door open. Contact the door gently so the impact does not cause your foot supports to go out of adjustment.
- Pay attention to the position of your feet, so you do not catch a toe. Catching your foot could twist your ankle or break your lower leg.
- Drive forward slowly, pushing the door open.

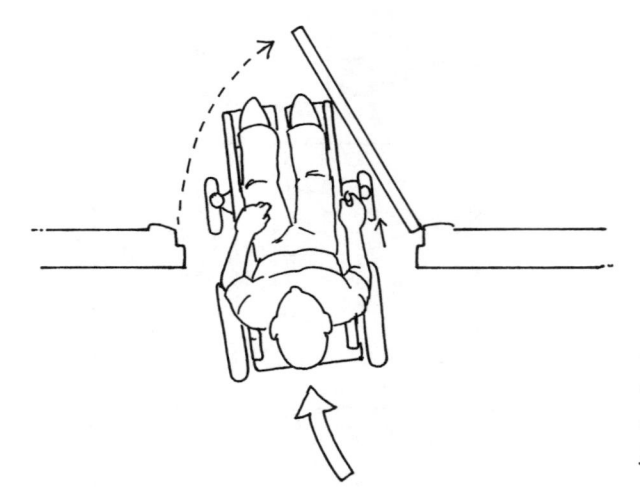

Push your foot supports against the kick plate to open a free-swinging door.

Doors that open away from you

- Turn slightly to the side as you reach the door. Reach to the side, unlatch the door, and open it.
- As the door swings open, turn your wheelchair so both casters touch the threshold. The ride will be smoother if both casters cross at the same time (See Section 3.2 for more information about crossing thresholds and other obstacles).
- If the door is spring-loaded, you may need to push the door with your hand as well as with your foot supports.

54

Section 3.3: Doorways and Tight Environments

- You may need to close the door after you go through it. If the door is not spring-loaded you can turn around and push the door closed with your wheelchair.

Doors that open toward you

- If the hinges are on the left, rotate your wheelchair slightly to the right as you approach the door. Reach to the left to unlatch and open the door.
- Pull the door open by backing up your wheelchair.
- As the door swings open, pivot your wheelchair to the left to block the door open with your footrests.
- Continue to move forward through the doorway. If the door is spring-loaded, it may begin to close, but if you are already on your way through, it will contact your back wheels and should not be a problem.

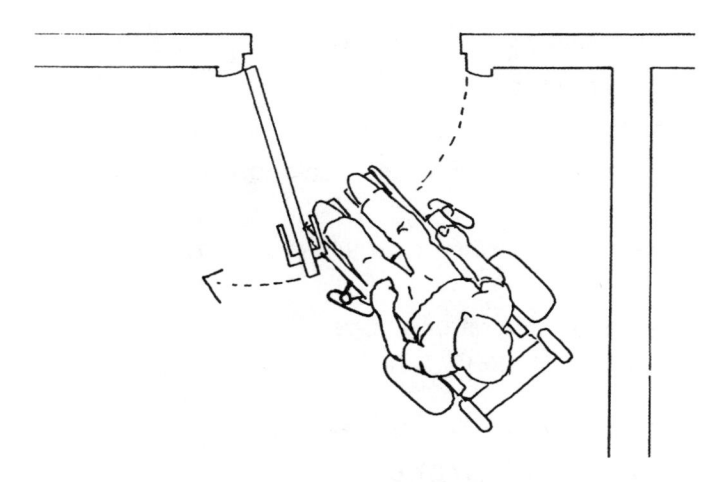

As the door swings open, pivot left to block the door open.

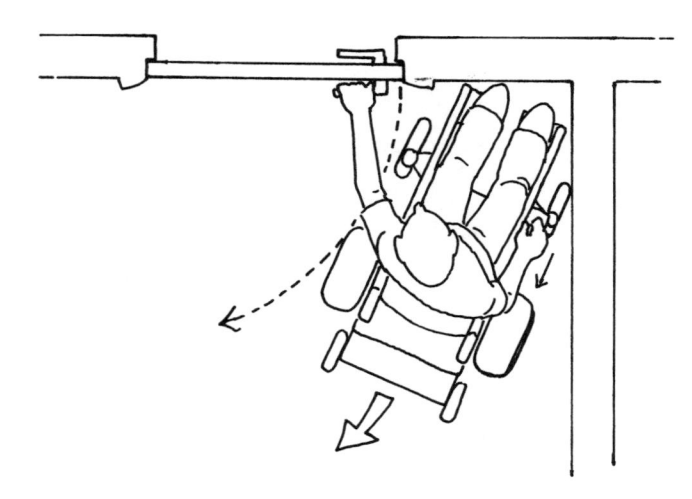

Pull the door open by backing up your wheelchair.

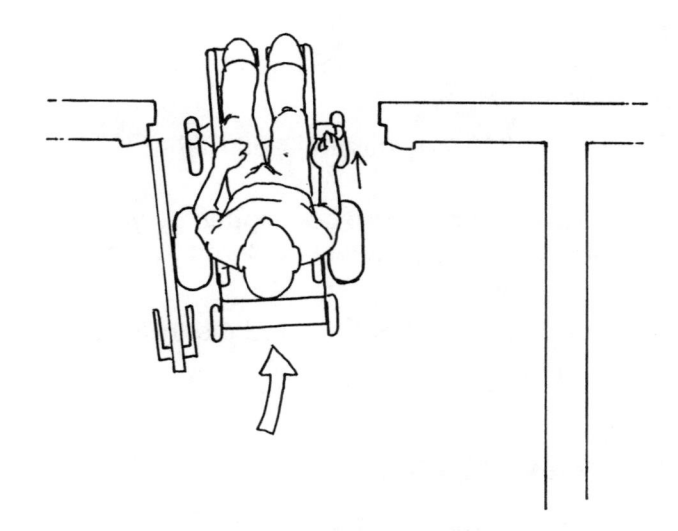

Then continue to move forward through the doorway.

55

Going forward through doors that open toward you with no clearance space

- Approach from the side opposite the door handle.
- Reach forward, unlatch the door and back up your wheelchair to pull the door open.
- While it is swinging open, drive your wheelchair into the doorway.
- A spring-loaded door may hit or scrape your wheelchair or your rear wheels as you go through.

Going backward through doors that open toward you with no clearance space

- Turn your wheelchair so your back is to the door.
- Reach behind you, unlatch the door and drive forward to pull the door open.
- When the door is open wide enough, hold on to the edge of the door to open it wider.
- Back up next to the door and continue backing through the doorway.
- The door may begin to close but it will be stopped by your wheelchair. If it prevents you from continuing through the doorway, push it open again.
- Keep moving backward until you have cleared the threshold and can turn forward again.

Manual Sliding Doors

Manual sliding doors slide instead of swinging open. Exterior sliding glass and screen doors usually slide on floor tracks. Floor tracks can be more difficult to cross than conventional thresholds because they are taller and have sharper edges (See Section 3.2 for more information about crossing thresholds and other obstacles). Drop-offs on one side of a floor threshold can be hazardous and can cause you to lose your balance.

"Pocket" sliding doors, usually found inside, ride on an overhead track and do not have a threshold to obstruct your passage. Indoor "pocket" doors should not present a problem once they are open because there is no threshold.

Practice sliding heavier doors with a spotter to prevent you from losing your balance.

- With a spotter nearby, practice with sliding glass or screen doors. Ask the spotter to stand to one side of the wheelchair, ready to catch your upper body if you should fall forward when reaching for the door handle.
- If the handle is on the right, rotate your wheelchair slightly to the right as you reach the door. Reach sideways to open the door with your left hand.
- Back up your wheelchair to pull the door open until it is wide enough to pass through.

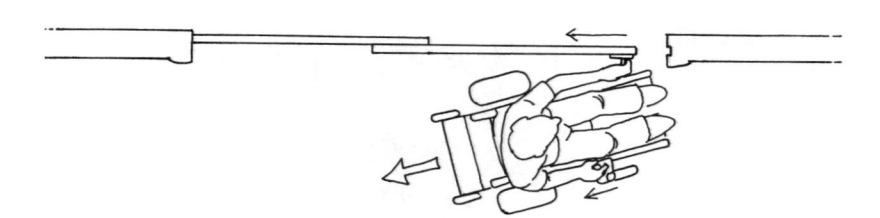

Hold on to the door handle as you back up your wheelchair to open or close the door.

- Reposition your wheelchair so both casters cross the threshold at the same time (see Section 3.2 for more information about crossing thresholds and obstacles).
- As you drive through, watch for a drop off on the outside of the track. A sudden drop may cause you to lose your balance and fall forward.
- After you pass through the doorway, rotate into a good position and use the power of your wheelchair to slide the door shut.

Doors in a Sequence

Many buildings, particularly in colder climates, have entrances with two doors in quick succession. There will typically be one swinging door, a short space, and then a second swinging door. If there is enough space for you to pass through the first door and reposition yourself for the second, you can follow the recommendations for passing through conventional swinging doors.

Problems arise when the doors are spaced so closely that you cannot pass all the way through the first door and into the space before you need to open the second. Problems also occur when one or both doors open toward you and take up your maneuvering room. As the doors swing, they create obstacles you must work to avoid.

Before attempting doors in a sequence, you should know how to open a single swinging door. Have a spotter nearby as you practice in case you get trapped between the doors. Hotels, post offices and other public buildings are good places to practice opening doors in sequence.

- Open the first door using the steps listed under "Manual Swinging Doors."
- If the second door opens into the space between the doors, and the space is short, try to use your wheelchair to prop the first door open. This will give you room to back up through the first doorway and position your wheelchair while you open and pass through the second doorway.

How to ask for assistance

- If opening the door (or doors) is difficult, ask someone to help you by opening and holding one or both of the doors for you to drive through.
- You may need to plan how to hold the first door open while your assistant changes position to open the second door.
- If you need help crossing the threshold, see Section 3.2.

Double-leaf Doors

A double-leaf door is made up of two narrow swinging doors that open in the center. Saloon-style and French doors are considered double-leaf doors. If each door is standard size, each half of the door is 32 inches wide. You might encounter double doors where both doors will need to be opened.

Double-leaf doors are fairly rare. However, if you spend a lot of time in a place with double-leaf doors, take some time to practice.

If the door handle is beyond your reach, ask a spotter to stand to one side of your wheelchair. The spotter should be ready to stabilize your upper body if you lose your balance while leaning forward to open the latch. If opening the door (or doors) is difficult, ask someone to hold one or both doors open as you drive through.

Open double-leaf doors using the skills for manual swinging doors. If you need help crossing the threshold, see Section 3.2.

Helpful Hints

If you have trouble using a particular door, look for an alternate entrance. You may need to ask someone familiar with the building. To avoid such situations, phone the establishment before your visit to inquire about access. Perhaps they can prop the doors open for you.

If the doors are at your home or workplace, look into having the doors powered to open electronically. A large button can be placed to allow you to push the button as you approach. Ideally, you will want to place the button well in advance of the door to allow the door to swing open before you get there.

Narrow Doors

To pass unassisted through a doorway too narrow for your wheelchair, you may have to do a series of transfers. Although it is usually easier to find a different route, you may have no choice but to attempt an entry. These situations usually arise in hotel rooms where the door to the bathroom is narrow and the bathroom space is small. First, you should try to find a room with a more accessible bathroom. If the bathroom with the narrow door is your only option, try to get the door removed from its hinges. Most hotels will remove the door for you. If the doorway is still too narrow for you to enter, your only choice may be to transfer into a chair that can then be slid into the bathroom with assistance. Many powered wheelchair users who need assistance in the bathroom travel with a collapsible shower chair.

Practice on doors of different widths that swing in different directions. When practicing, have a spotter there to assist if you get stuck and need help.

Entering with a chair

- Put a four-legged chair near the doorway.
- Transfer independently or get assistance transferring into the chair. Have your assistant pull the chair backward so that your legs follow you while you hold on to the chair.

How a spotter can help

- Help the wheelchair rider practice manipulating the wheelchair through tight doorways.
- Be available to assist with a transfer if necessary.
- Be available to assist with a "transfer" chair.

Automatic Doors

Automatic doors are usually found at grocery stores and medical facilities. Automatic doors are very convenient, since they do the work of opening the door for you. Some automatic doors are operated by stepping or driving onto a sensor pad that is slightly higher than the ground.

Many automatic doors are triggered by an optical sensor aimed at an area in front of the door. If a person enters the area scanned by the sensor, the door opens. If the door does not open, look around the door frame for an optical sensor. Approach the door again, this time crossing the path of the sensor. Waving your hand or arm above your head can trigger optical sensors to open the door.

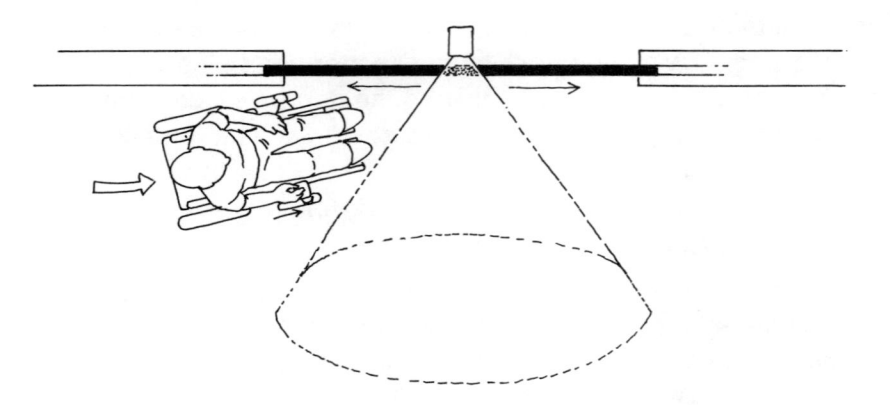

Place yourself and your wheelchair in the area that the sensor "sees" so that the automatic door will open.

You may be moving faster than a person who is walking when you approach an automatic door. Slow to "walking speed" to give the door time to swing or slide open.

- While these doors are designed to stay open as you pass through, some sensors and timing devices may still cause the doors to close on you.

Revolving Doors and Turnstiles

An alternative entrance should be offered in places with revolving doors and turnstiles. If an alternative entrance is not available, you may have to negotiate the revolving door or turnstile to enter the building.

In many places, the door attendant can fold the revolving doors flat to create a conventional entrance. If not, watch a few revolutions of the revolving doors to get a sense of the timing required to use them. Closely examine the space available between the sections of the revolving doors to determine if your wheelchair will fit or if you might get stuck. Ask an assistant to slowly rotate the doors so you can concentrate on driving your wheelchair.

While revolving doors that rotate in a large oval may be able to accommodate wheelchairs, exercise caution before using them.

Turnstiles that can be opened like gates should not pose a problem for you. But if the turnstile cannot be operated like a gate, and the arms lock in each position, you could get trapped.

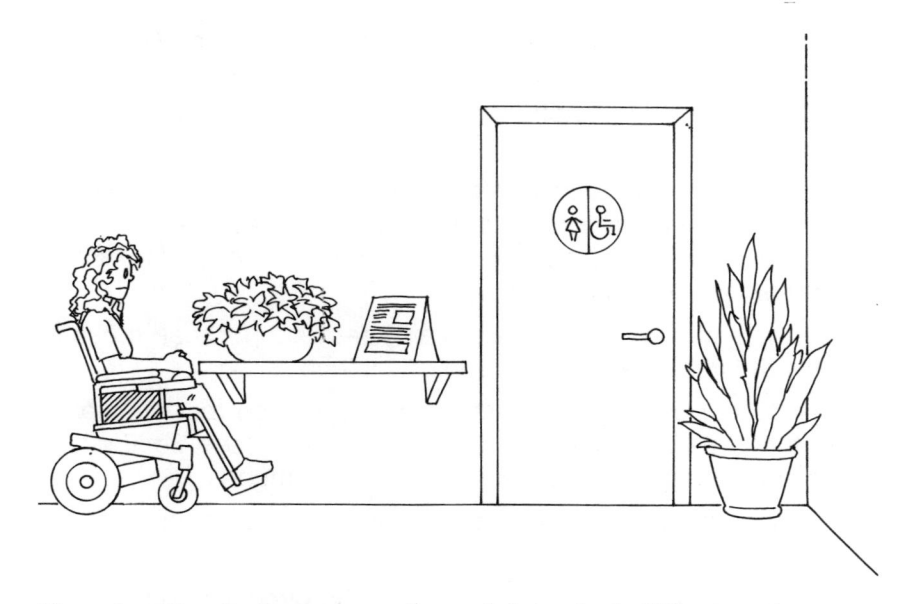

Obstacles often limit access to doors. Inform the building's management so they will refrain from placing objects near doors in the future.

Doors with Objects Around Them

Although the Americans with Disabilities Act Accessibility Guidelines require doors to have a certain amount of clear space around them, obstacles such as trash cans, free-standing signs, ashtrays and potted plants are frequently found alongside doors. These obstacles can make reaching the door handle and opening and closing the door difficult. Ways to cope with such objects include:

- Push the obstacles out of the way with your foot supports.
- Ask someone to move the obstacle for you.
- Inform the management of the business. They may not have recognized the problem and most likely will be willing to correct it.

Helpful Hints

If you have trouble using a particular door, find an alternate route. You may need to ask someone more familiar with the building. Though searching for an alternate door may be inconvenient at the time, it will save a lot of time in the future. The next time you visit that building, you will already know where the best path of travel is.

Tight Environments

A lack of floor space, objects on walls, and protruding furniture such as tables can all limit your maneuvering space. Places such as narrow hallways, small vans, small apartments, and household bathrooms can leave you with very little room to move. Because it can be difficult to use a wheelchair in tight environments, it is often a good idea to find alternative routes or spaces to use.

- Remember that you can move the front portion of your wheelchair closer to certain objects, such as under bathroom sinks or near toilets, because of the smaller front casters and lower front end. Look underneath to be sure your knees or legs will not contact any sharp edges.
- The height of your rear wheels and back support can make it difficult for you to back up to many objects.
- Remember that your casters must be in the correct orientation for the front of the chair to change directions (see Section 2.5 for more information about caster management).
- Backing into a small space often puts you in a better position to maneuver once inside.
- Removing the foot supports reduces the overall length of the wheelchair and might make it easier to turn around. Driving backward can prevent you from driving over your feet. Be careful not to bump your feet or get them caught in your casters. Removing one foot support and crossing that foot over the opposite ankle may also help you maneuver in a tight space.

Backing up

- Drive your wheelchair backward until you reach a space wide enough for you to be able to turn around.
- Be sure to look behind you for other people or obstacles.

Three-point turns

- Make sure the pathway is a little wider than the length of your wheelchair.
- Check for approaching people and obstacles behind you.
- If the path is clear, pull to one side of the pathway.
- Turn the chair sharply and drive slowly toward the opposite side of the path.

- When you cannot go any farther forward, back up, turning in the opposite direction.
- When you cannot go any farther back, go forward, again turning in the opposite direction.
- Continue moving back and forth to complete the turn.

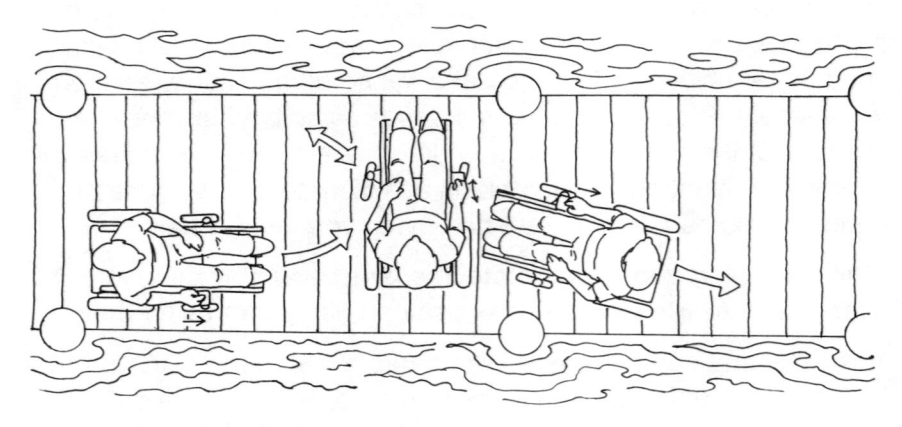

In tight spaces, you might be able to make the turn in steps by moving back and forth. Although called a three-point turn, this maneuver may actually take more than three movements to complete the turn.

Turning into a doorway from a narrow hallway

When turning into a doorway from a narrow hallway using a **rear-wheel drive** chair, drive along the far side of the hallway before starting the turn.

When using a **front-wheel drive** chair, you may need to drive along the wall closest to the door opening. The space in the hallway behind you will permit you to turn into the doorway without hitting the wall behind you.

In a **mid-wheel drive** chair, you will want to drive down the center of the hallway and pivot in front of the doorway to turn and drive through it. Mid-wheel drive chairs offer intuitive maneuverability,

Section 3.3: Doorways and Tight Environments

allowing you to drive to the center of the doorway and make a sharp turn into the doorway.

If you are turning from a narrow hallway into a narrow doorway, you may not have enough room. Sometimes removing one of the foot supports will allow you to make this maneuver. To do this, cross the leg without the foot support over the leg with the foot support and then fold up or remove the empty foot support.

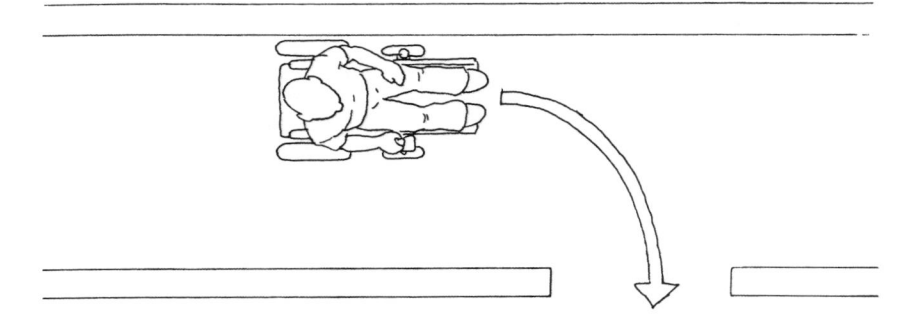

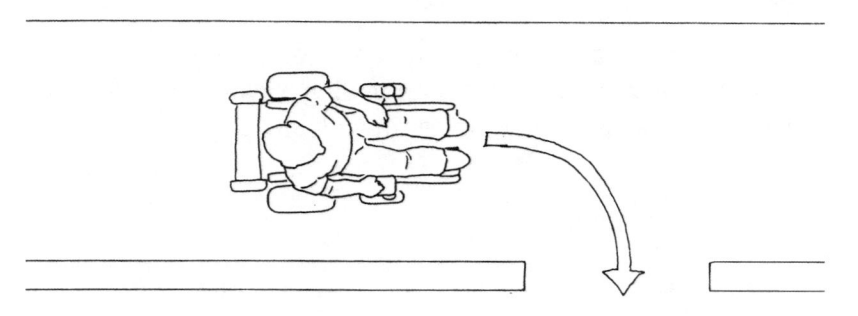

A mid-wheel drive chair pivots at the user's body, making turns a bit more intuitive.

In a rear-wheel drive chair, making as wide a turn as possible will help you turn through a doorway in a narrow hall.

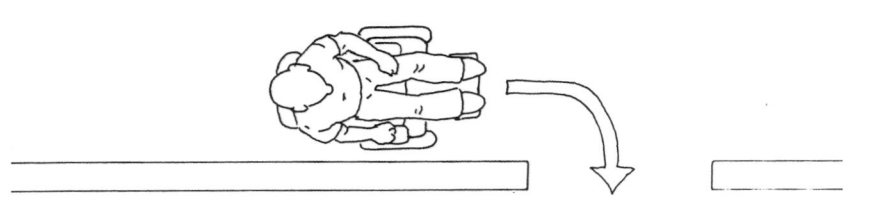

Helpful Hints

If convenient or possible, consider using a manual wheelchair with assistance as a back-up when you know that you are going to a place where it will be difficult to move around in your powered wheelchair.

In a front-wheel drive chair, the rear end of the chair swings out behind you when turning. To allow room for this, track close to where you will turn.

Vans

Depending on the location of your drive wheels, you may find that backing onto your van lift (rather than driving forward onto it) may allow greater maneuverability inside the vehicle.

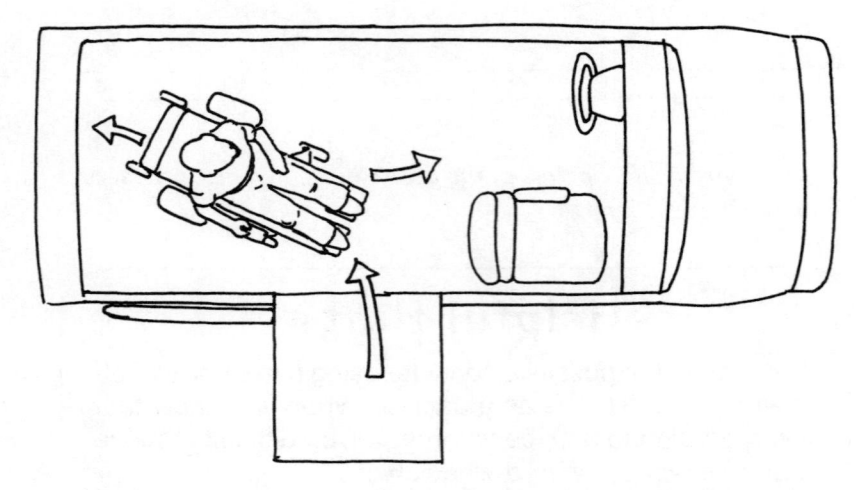

In some situations, backing in may make it easier to maneuver. This person is able to back into the van and reach the driver's area without hitting the sidewall.

Section 3.4

Rough Terrain

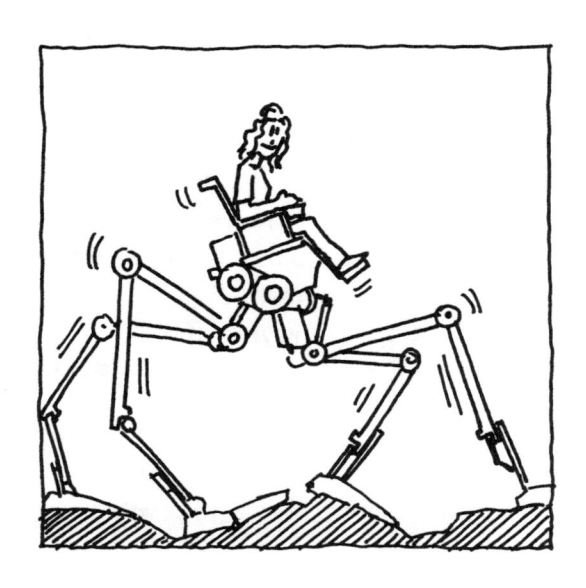

If you're active outdoors, you will encounter many surfaces that are difficult to negotiate in your wheelcBefore attempting to learn rough terrain skills, you should be able to drive a wheelchair forward and backward and maintain balance and control when driving over thresholds.

Larger, softer and wider tires make travel over rough surfaces and obstacles easier, but can be sluggish and can reduce the distance you can travel between battery charges on smooth surfaces, such as concrete or vinyl flooring. Section 2.5 discusses how tires affect performance.

Practice crossing different surfaces with assistance to get a feel for how rough a surface you can negotiate alone. If bumps on rough terrain jolt you out of position, stop to reposition yourself before you get out of control. Traveling slower may improve the ride.

When learning to travel across rough terrain, have a spotter there to assist as necessary. Practice on rough tile, working up to hard, uneven surfaces, such as buckled sidewalks, and finally attempting softer surfaces, such as grass or gravel. Progress slowly over any new surface at first. There may be an optimum speed that is fast enough for momentum to help carry you over the rough surface but slow enough to maintain balance and control.

Hard, Uneven Surfaces

Look at the surface to see what obstacles you may encounter. Be aware of obstacles such as grooves between tiles that may catch your tires, throw rugs that can tangle in your casters, and changes in surface type. The living room carpet transition to kitchen vinyl flooring, could throw you off balance.

Move across the wooden planks of decks, piers and boardwalks perpendicular to the boards so your casters will not get stuck in the spaces between the boards. When surfaces change, such as when vinyl flooring transitions to carpet, a small step may exist. Crossing at a 45 to 90 degree angle will make this type of transition easier. To avoid catching your casters in tiles, try crossing perpendicular or at least diagonal to the grooves.

Be aware that riding over bumps can trigger muscle spasms. Extensor spasms can make it difficult to stay upright and balanced in your chair. If you

Chapter Three: Navigational Skills

have spasticity you will learn what types of terrain will trigger the spasms. Some people use Velcro™ on their shoes or bungee cords to keep their feet on their foot supports.

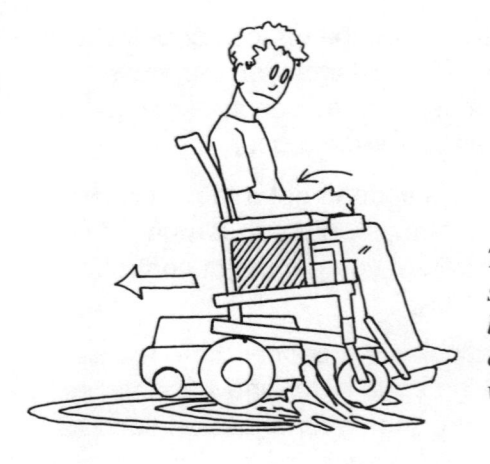

Throw rugs and area rugs not secured to the floor often slide, bunch and can get under your chair. Remove or avoid them whenever possible.

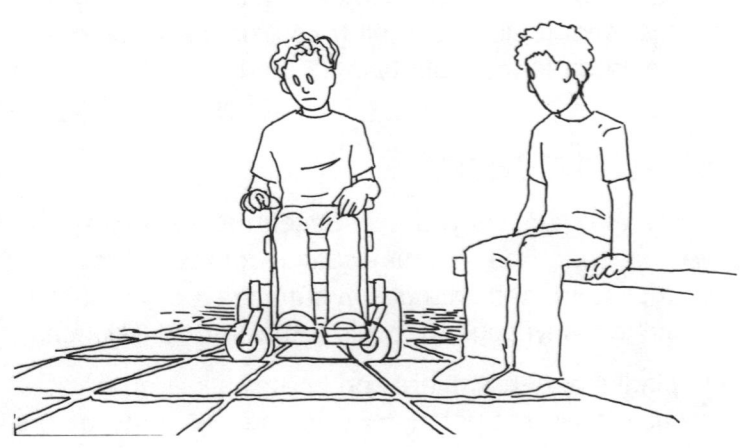

Sometimes the space between tiles is deep and wide enough for your casters to get caught.

Soft Surfaces

Be sure to maintain forward momentum when crossing soft surfaces such as gravel, mud, sand and clay. Moving slowly or stopping on soft surfaces can cause your wheelchair to sink into the surface.

Practice crossing different soft surfaces with a spotter, progressing from grass and shallow mud to sand. Keep your casters aligned in the same direction, as they will not rotate on soft terrain (see Section 2.5 for more information about caster management). Have a spotter walk on your non-joystick side, ready to keep you from falling forward in your wheelchair if your chair stops suddenly.

On a soft surface, pushing forward on the back of the chair can force the front casters into the surface. Pushing down on the push handles can relieve weight from the casters and increase traction on the rear wheels. However, this further weights the rear wheels down into the surface.

Crossing rough terrain with assistance

If you think you will need help to cross an uneven or soft surface, ask someone to assist you.

- Ask the assistant to walk on the non-joystick side of your wheelchair.
- As the assistant pushes, drive your wheelchair slowly forward.
- Ask the assistant to prevent you from falling forward in the chair if you lose your balance or if the chair stops suddenly.
- Ask the assistant to stand next to the wheelchair to help pull as needed on the front of the arm support or leg support. On some wheelchairs, the arm supports may not lock into place and they will just pull out.
- If the wheelchair gets stuck, have an assistant use a belt or a piece of webbing to pull up on the front of the wheelchair. This will help keep the front casters from digging into the surface.

The strap must be attached to a secure and strong part of the wheelchair. Attaching a strap to the frame near the front wheel is a good place to start. You can have a second person push from behind.

In a rear-wheel drive chair, driving backward on the surface may work better than driving forward. An assistant can push on the front of the wheelchair in this case. Front-wheel drive chairs often drive better on soft surfaces. Laying a mat or scraps of wood or branches on the surface can help you get out of a difficult, isolated trouble spot.

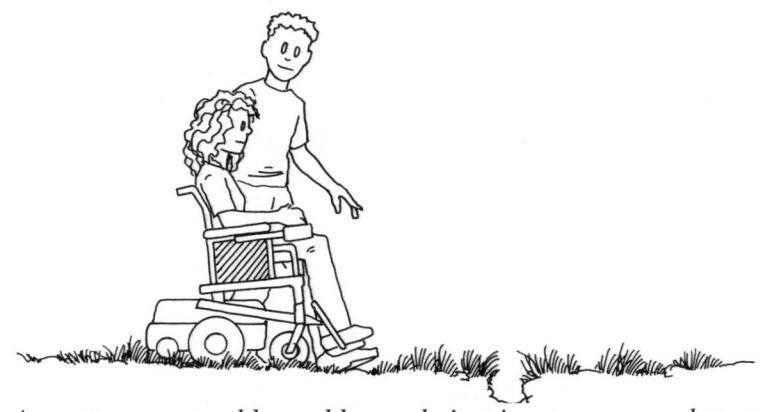

A spotter can stand by and be ready just in case you need some help maintaining your balance.

Section 3.5

Ramps

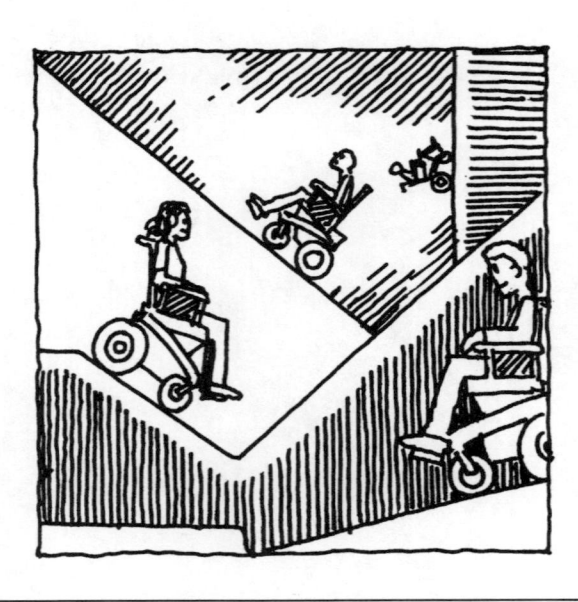

According to the Americans with Disabilities Act (ADA) Accessibility Guidelines, a standard ramp in the built environment should have a grade no steeper than 1:12. This means that for every inch of rise (change in height), there should be 12 inches of run (change in length). This is sometimes referred to as an 8 percent grade or slope. Using this formula, a ramp going to a door with two 8-inch steps should be at least 16 feet long.

A standard ramp is gradual enough for powered wheelchairs to climb safely, but the limit beyond that is different for each powered wheelchair.

With experimentation, you will learn how steep a ramp you can negotiate without assistance. Always use a spotter when practicing on ramps and when driving up a steeper ramp for the first time. Practice descending steep ramps with a spotter until you find one that is at the limit of your trunk stability. Experience the loss of stability, and remember the steepness of the slope that caused this to happen. When climbing steeper ramps you may reach a point where you will begin to tip to the rear or the wheelchair may just run out of power. Obtain assistance before going up or down slopes this steep, or steeper, in the future. Loading docks are good places to find steeper than normal ramps for practice on steep ramps.

Going Up a Ramp

- There will be a tendency for the wheelchair to tip backward when driving up a steep ramp. A backpack or other gear on the back of your wheelchair will cause you to tip backward more easily. If you use a reclining back wheelchair or a tilt-in-space seating system, you will find that having your back support in the fully upright position gives you the greatest stability when driving up a ramp.
- Drive slowly to maintain control.
- On steep ramps, it is best to keep a straight path. Approaching a steep ramp at an angle will increase the severity of the cross slope. Cross slopes are discussed later in this section.

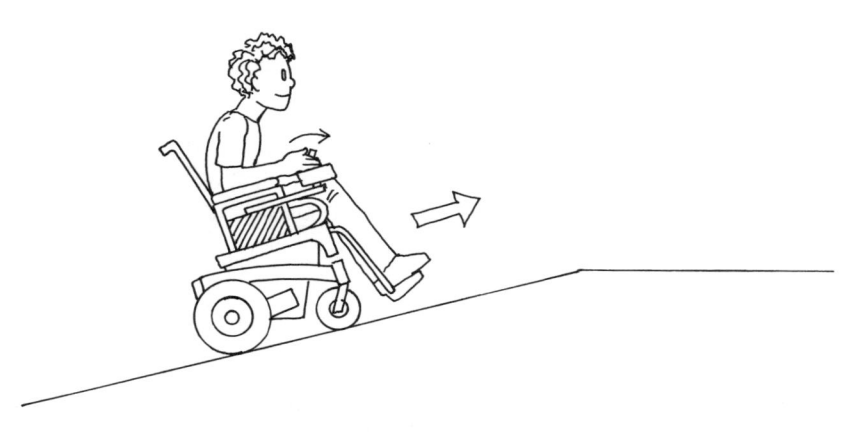

Lean forward when you are going up a steep ramp facing forward.

How a spotter can help

- Walk behind the wheelchair and place your hands close to the push handles or back posts. Try not to influence the movement of the wheelchair.
- Prevent the front casters from lifting off the ground by lifting up or by pushing forward on the push handles or back support.
- If the wheelchair runs out of power, assist by pushing the wheelchair up the slope.

Going Down a Ramp

Before descending a ramp, always check for obstacles such as cracks and changes in level. Also examine the base of the ramp for obstacles you may need to cross, such as drainage grates.

Always shift your weight back when going down ramps, and proceed slowly to maintain control. As you get more comfortable and confident with ramps, you will be able to increase your speed and remain safe.

Be careful of foot support clearance when you get to the base of the ramp. Drive slowly in case your foot supports contact the ground. If they do, you will come to an abrupt stop.

Always practice descending ramps with a spotter. Travel down ramps of increasing steepness until you find the angle where you can no longer descend the ramp alone with confidence. Always obtain assistance when you do not feel comfortable descending a ramp independently.

Practice with a spotter on the non-joystick side of your wheelchair, ready to catch your upper body if you should fall forward.

Going down a ramp forward independently

- Examine the ramp for obstacles.
- Drive slowly to maintain control.
- The ramp may be so steep that you will lose forward balance. If this happens, compensate by shifting your weight back (see Section 2.3 for more information about shifting your weight).
- Putting the joystick in reverse can further slow the speed of some chairs. However, this technique is not recommended for wheelchairs with non-digital controllers on a continuous basis, as the braking action could permanently damage the controller or motors.
- Some ramps might be so steep that you will lose traction under the rear wheels and begin to slide. You will maintain more control by driving forward than you will sliding forward.

Chapter Three: Navigational Skills

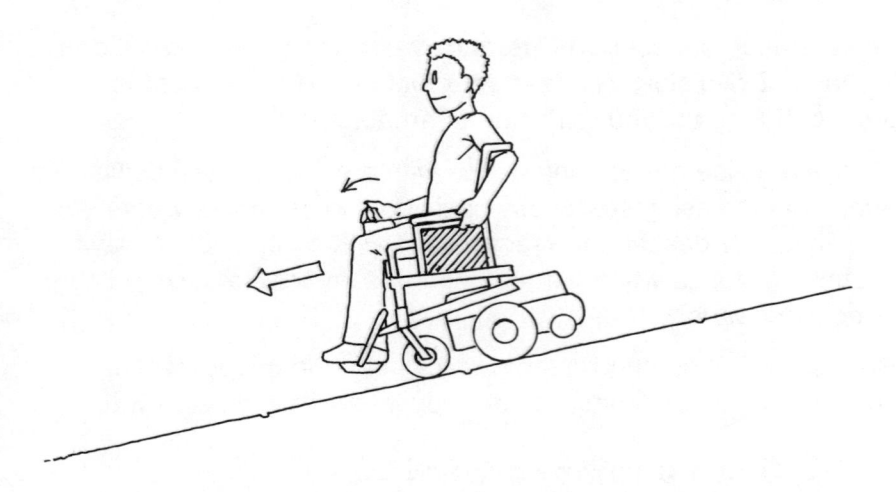

Hooking one arm around a push handle and leaning back into your back support may help you keep your balance when going down ramps.

How a spotter can help

- Walk on the non-joystick side of the wheelchair rider as the rider moves down the ramp.
- Be ready to catch the wheelchair rider's upper body if the rider falls forward.
- Stand behind the wheelchair rider and reach over the shoulder to provide additional trunk support.

Going down a ramp backward independently

Traveling down a steep ramp can cause you to lose trunk stability in the forward direction. When shifting your weight back during the descent or hooking your elbow on the push handle is not enough to maintain your balance, descend the ramp backward. You should also descend a ramp backward if you believe it is so steep that the foot supports will hit the ground at the bottom.

- Check the ramp for any obstacles.
- Move slowly to maintain control.

- It may be difficult to maintain the direction you want to go when you are driving backward down a ramp. Have a spotter or an assistant ready to help guide the wheelchair from the rear.
- If you are using anti-tippers, watch for clearance of the anti-tippers at the bottom of the ramp. If your anti-tippers get caught at the bottom of the ramp, you could tip over backwards.
- Letting go of the joystick should cause the wheelchair to dynamically brake and slow or stop.

How a spotter can help

- Walk on the non-joystick side of the wheelchair and hold on to the wheelchair frame to physically assist with guiding the wheelchair straight.
- If the ramp is steep, position yourself behind the wheelchair, hold the push handles, and walk backward down the ramp. Move with the wheelchair as it drives backward.

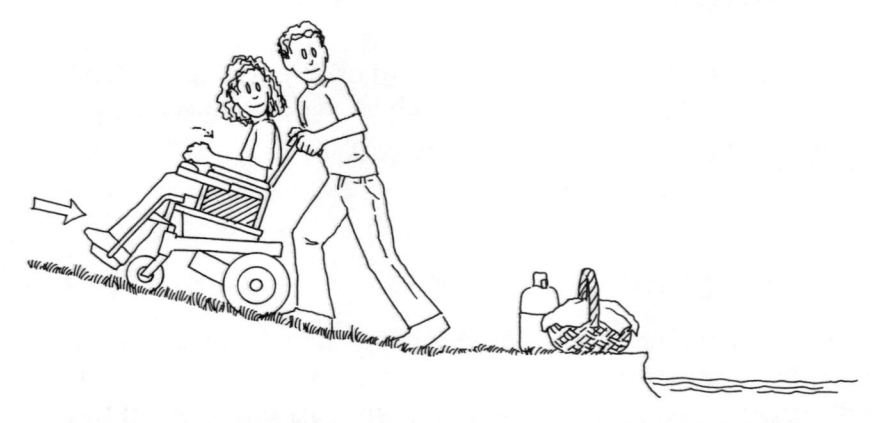

To slow the wheelchair, a spotter can walk behind the wheelchair with his or her hands on the push handles, leaning forward into the back support.

Very Steep Ramps

If the ramp is too steep for your wheelchair to ascend or descend, even with an assistant, find an alternate route or have two or three assistants help you by pushing and/or pulling.

- Attach pull straps to the wheelchair near the front casters to enable helpers to pull on the left and right sides of the wheelchair. Have the strongest assistant behind the wheelchair assist by pushing.
- You can assist by driving the wheelchair slowly to apply as much power as possible.
- When going down, applying a very small amount of reverse power will keep the parking brakes from engaging. You will also be able to assist with steering. If this does not work, disengage the drive motors and have your assistant(s) manually roll the chair down.

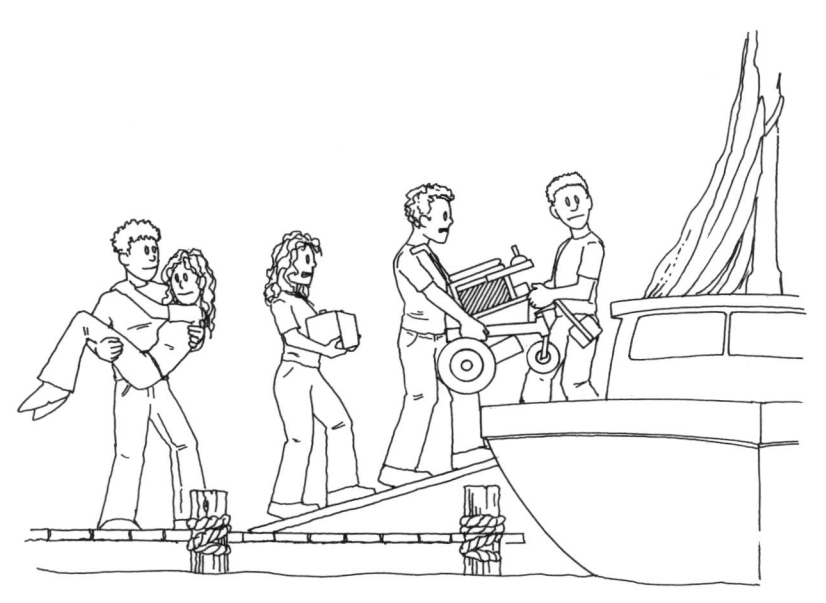

If the ramp is too steep or narrow, have your assistant transport you and your wheelchair separately.

How a spotter can help

- Walk behind the wheelchair rider as the rider moves up the ramp with your hands near the push handles. If necessary, push the wheelchair to keep the casters from lifting off the ground, and to provide extra power to ascend the ramp or to slow the descent.
- The second spotter should walk on the joystick side of the wheelchair rider as they move up or down the ramp. Be prepared to shut the wheelchair off if there are any difficulties.

Telescoping or Portable Ramps

Telescoping or portable ramps are made so that they can be moved and used in different locations. Sometimes the ramp is wide enough for the whole wheelchair to fit on it. Other times, two narrow ramps are used under the wheels on each side. If these narrow ramps are used, make sure they are wide enough for your wheels. Some wheelchairs are made so the casters are not in line with the main wheels. If this is the case with your wheelchair, you may have more difficulty using portable ramps because individually they may not be wide enough for both the front and rear wheels. Before using telescoping or portable ramps:

- Stretch the ramps out on a flat surface and be sure your wheels can safely drive through the full length of the ramps before attempting to use them on an incline.

Turning Around on a Ramp

The safest way to turn around on a ramp is to continue traveling until you reach a level resting area or the end of the ramp. However, this is not always possible. For example, you might be driving on a road or trail that is a steep ramp. With a little practice, you will be able to turn around on a ramp safely. Lean and shift your weight in the uphill direction as you turn. This helps to move the center of mass uphill and will help to prevent your wheelchair from tipping.

Chapter Three: Navigational Skills

How to turn around on a ramp

- Look behind you to check for oncoming traffic.
- If the path is clear, move to the non-joystick side of the ramp and stop.
- When you have come to a halt, turn your wheelchair in the direction of the joystick until you are sideways on the ramp. This allows you to maintain your upper body position with your joystick arm. You may find it easier to turn in the other direction if you have more ability to balance with the other arm.
- Keep your weight shifted uphill.
- Continue to turn your wheelchair using the joystick until you are facing downhill. Be sure to keep your weight shifted back.
- Drive your wheelchair forward down the ramp.

Note: It will be important for you to determine the steepest ramp on which you can ascend, descend, and turn around. Always have a spotter with you when determining the maximum limits of your wheelchair.

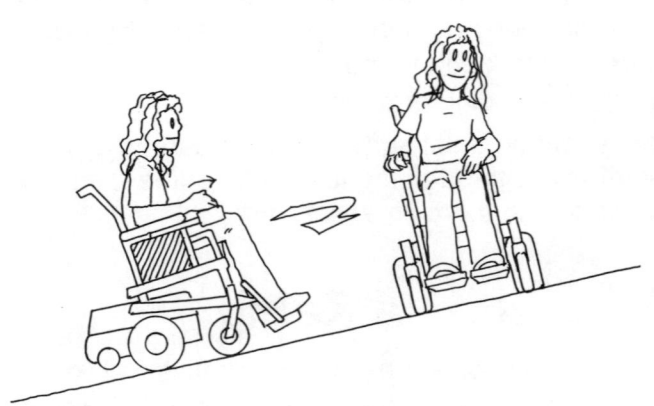

When you make a turn on a ramp, be careful that your wheelchair does not tip sideways.

How a spotter can help

- Stand downhill from the rider throughout the turn to keep the rider from falling forward out of the chair and to keep the chair from tipping.

Grade Transitions

Curb ramps are, unfortunately, often built up to or beyond the maximum slope allowance (8.3%), and at the bottom of the curb ramp the gutter slopes up in the opposite direction toward the center of the street. This creates a downslope-to-upslope transition where the foot supports can dig into the ramp or the gutter, bringing the wheelchair to an abrupt stop. This can cause you to be thrown forward in the chair or completely out of the chair if you do not use a lap belt.

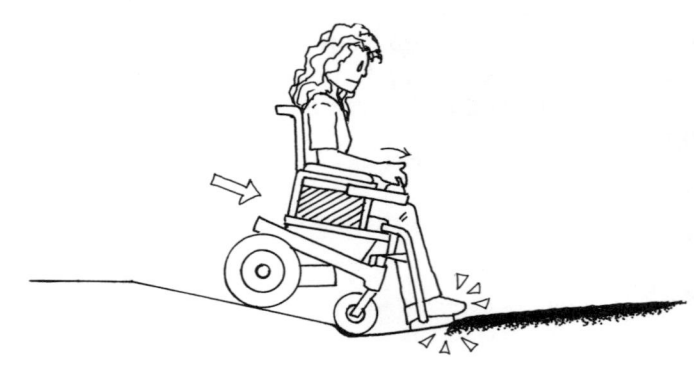

Foot supports that are adjusted too low can get caught going through a curb ramp.

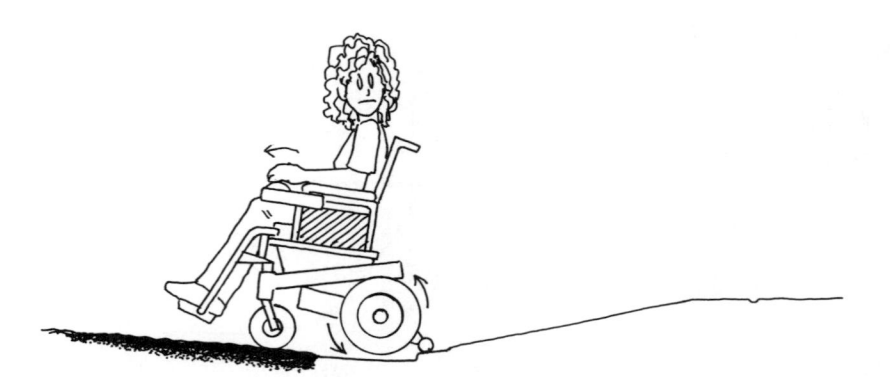

Anti-tip wheels can get caught where there is a lip at the base of the curb ramp and the ramp and gutter slopes create a rapidly changing grade.

Section 3.6

Cross Slopes

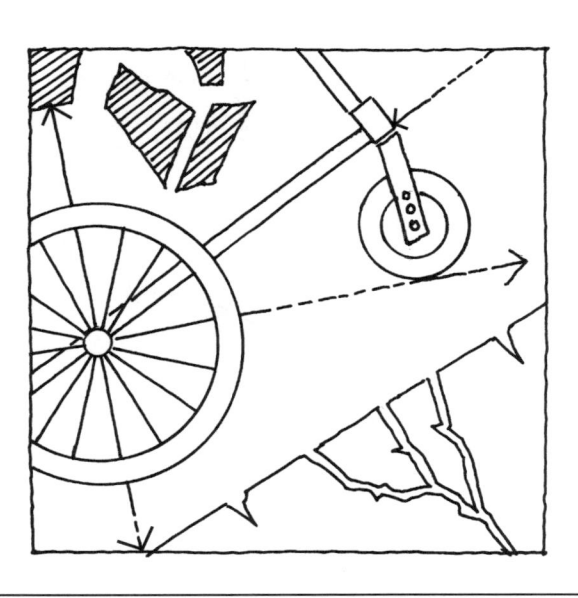

A cross slope or side slope is the slant a walkway has from side to side. Sidewalks are made with side slopes built in so that when it rains, the water flows to the curb and gutter. Built environments meeting ADA accessibility standards are not supposed to have a cross slope steeper than 2%. In the outdoor built environment it is quite common to encounter sidewalks with cross slopes in the 3-5% range. Even steeper side slopes occur in places where you must drive across a curb ramp or driveway crossing. When you must turn around on a standard ramp you will be on an 8% cross slope. Cross slopes also occur whenever you travel across a hill at an angle rather than straight up and down.

The experience of moving on a walkway with any side slope will be different for everyone depending on many factors, including, but not limited to, trunk stability, the type of surface, and the type of wheelchair that you use. Rear-wheel drive chairs tend to turn downhill on a cross slope, front-wheel drive chairs tend to turn uphill. Mid-wheel drive chairs, if properly adjusted, don't turn up or downhill. Many wheelchairs, especially rear-wheel drive chairs, will tend to roll in the downhill direction and you will have to compensate with the controls by correcting in the uphill direction. The steeper the side slope the more you may have to correct. A severe cross slope could cause your wheelchair to tip sideways. Remember to lean uphill to shift your center of mass and to help keep from tipping.

Walkways and Hills with Cross Slopes

- Always keep your body balanced by leaning in the uphill direction.
- Move forward at a speed that is less than full speed. You will have more directional control at a lower speed than if you try to travel at full speed.
- If there is a walkway or path, keep your wheelchair centered on it. This way, if you start to turn downhill, you will have room to make a correction. You will also have room to travel in the uphill direction if there is an obstacle you want to avoid.
- Driveway crossings can create nasty cross slopes. Make sure your wheelchair does not tip or veer sideways when you transition onto or off of a driveway crossing. Driveway crossings can create cross slopes of 8 to 15 percent or more.

How a spotter can help

- Walk on the downhill side to prevent the rider from losing balance.

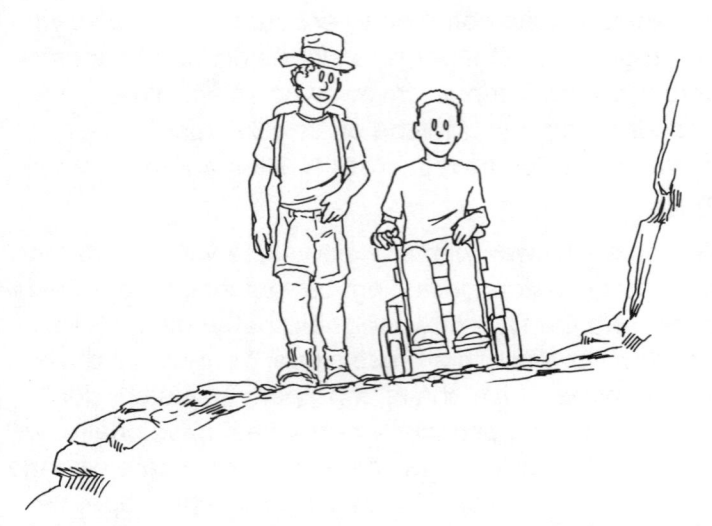

Have your spotter walk on the downhill side so if your wheelchair starts to turn or tip, the spotter can more easily assist you.

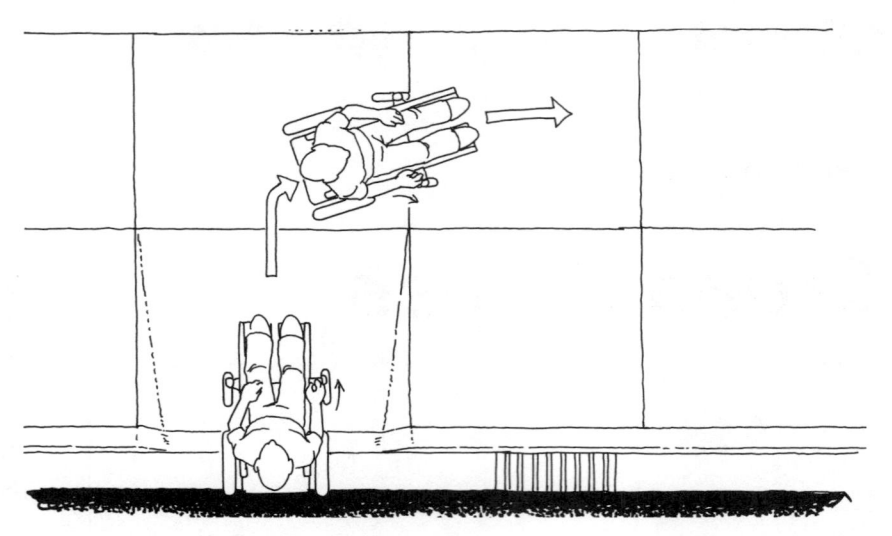

Curb ramps should have level landings at the top to prevent you from having to cross over the flares on the side of the ramp.

Curb Ramps

A curb ramp is a ramp with flared edges to allow you to get onto or off of the street. Curb ramps are often referred to as curb cuts. Diagonal curb ramps cut corners, creating cross slopes that must be negotiated.

If a side slope is too severe for you to safely drive across, the only alternative is to find another route. Some people find that they have to drive down the curb ramp into the street, then turn around, and then go back up the ramp to continue on their way.

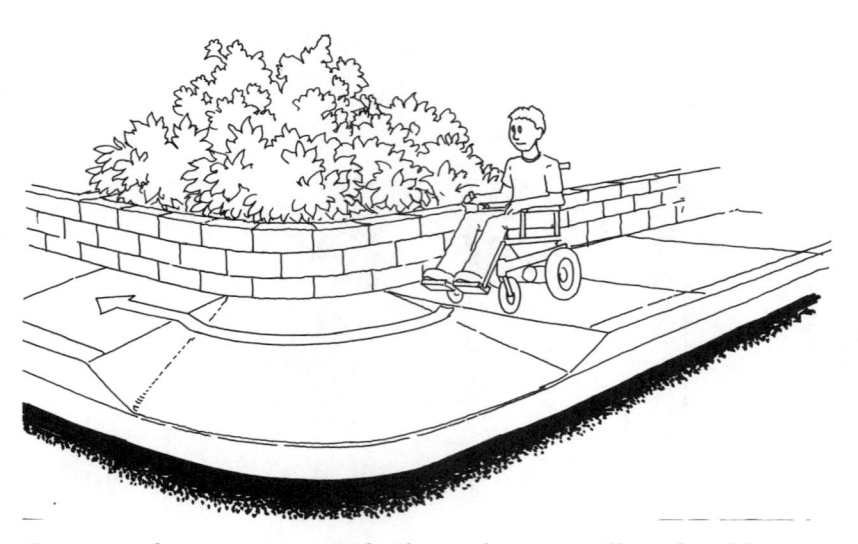

Corner curb ramps create side slopes that you will not be able to avoid and require you to cross the flares on the side of the ramp.

> ## Helpful Hints
>
> A wider wheel base results in a less "tippy" wheelchair when negotiating a side slope. However, a longer and wider wheel base also means a wider turning radius, and more space will be needed to turn the wheelchair around.
>
> Maneuvering in tight environments will be more difficult in a wider wheelchair as well.

When the sidewalk is immediately adjacent to the roadway, there is no room for a median between the sidewalk and the curb, so the full width of the sidewalk ends up being part of the curb ramp. This will cause you to have to drive across the top of the curb ramp and across the flares of the ramp. This can be a hazardous situation where one or more wheels can come off the ground, causing you to veer in the downhill direction.

How a spotter can help

- Position yourself on the downhill side of the wheelchair rider.
- You are in a position to prevent the wheelchair rider from losing balance or from veering into the street.

Driveway Crossings

Driveway crossings create cross slopes that you may not be able to avoid. Ideally, you should drive around the top of them, but this is not always possible.

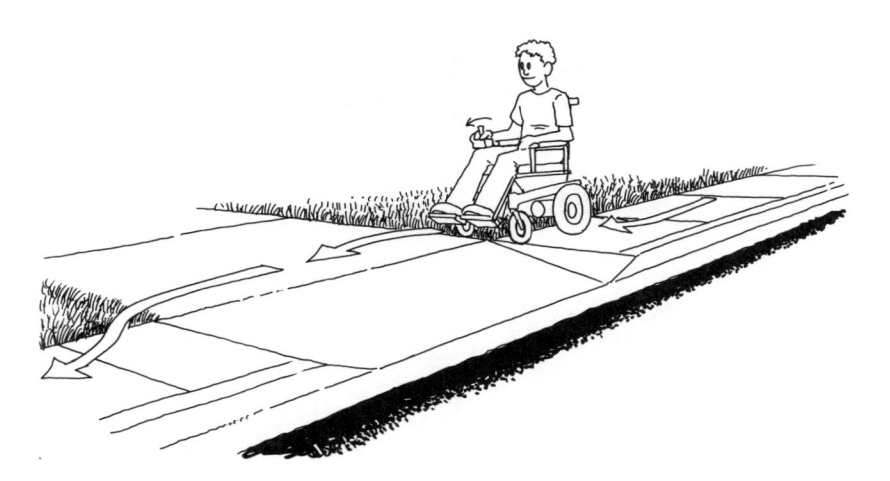

Driveway crossings also create side slopes. If you have to cross them, practice first with a spotter to make sure your wheelchair does not tip sideways.

Chapter Three: Navigational Skills

Section 3.7

Curbs and Steps

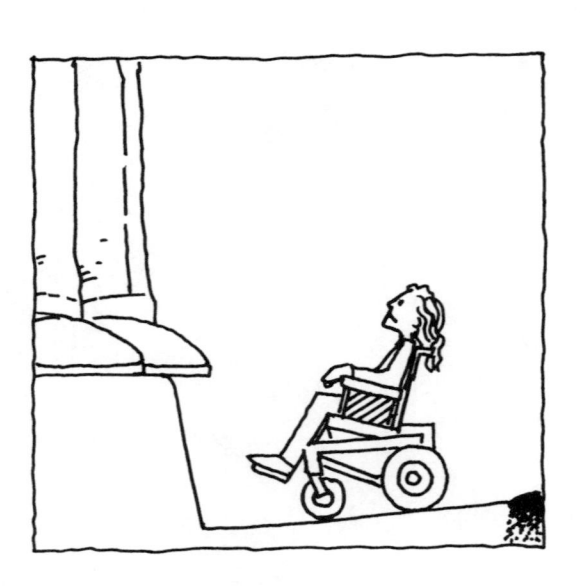

Curbs are the transition point between sidewalks and streets. If curb ramps are missing, in poor repair, or blocked, you will have to go up or down the curb. The lower the curb, the easier it is to negotiate. Depending on the type of chair you have, and with practice, you may be able to go up and down fairly high curbs. Some newer technology wheelchairs are designed to go up and down curbs. Some chairs can even go up and down curbs in the 3 to 6 inch range.

The skills in this section require a significant amount of wheelchair experience to accomplish, and may expose you and any assistants helping you to physical strain and serious injury. Always learn new skills with a RESNA certified Assistive Technology Practitioner or Supplier. Recognize the inherent danger and risk of performing these techniques. Realize that some obstacles you may never be able to safely negotiate with or without assistance.

When learning the techniques in this chapter, practice on curbs or single steps in quiet residential areas and avoid busy streets. Practice with a spotter until you can safely and consistently go up and down curbs. Climb increasingly higher curbs or single steps with a spotter to determine the highest curb you can handle independently.

Going Up Curbs or Steps

In the presence of a spotter, climb increasingly higher curbs to determine the maximum curb height you can go up independently. Your foot support clearance will determine the maximum curb height you can climb. If a curb is higher than your foot supports, you will need assistance to climb the curb or will need to find an alternate route. Almost all wheelchairs have to tip back to climb a curb when driving forward. Anti-tippers will significantly limit your ability to climb a curb in the forward direction because you will not be able to tip your wheelchair back very far. Anti-tippers will also limit your ability to climb a curb while driving backward because they will catch on curbs that are higher than the anti-tippers. Another consideration when going up curbs in your powered wheelchair is the clearance underneath your wheelchair between the front and rear wheels. Backing down a curb that is higher than your ground clearance may cause you to get stuck.

Going up curbs forward independently

- Check your anti-tipper clearance. The anti-tippers may keep you from tipping back far enough. If so, you will need assistance to reposition the anti-tippers or remove them for this maneuver.
- Also, Check your foot support clearance. If your foot supports do not clear the curb, you will need assistance.
- Ask your spotter to stand behind the wheelchair and prevent you from tipping backward.
- Slowly approach the curb in the forward direction until both front casters are touching the curb.
- Lean back as much as possible and drive the wheelchair forward until your front casters are up on the curb.
- Continue driving forward as you lean forward until the rear wheels are on the curb.
- You must transition the curb perpendicular at a 90 degree angle. If one of your main drive wheels climbs the curb before the other, your wheelchair can tip over to the side.
- After completing the maneuver, have your spotter reposition the anti-tippers or reinstall them on your chair.

How a spotter can help

- Check the anti-tipper clearance. If necessary, remove or reposition the anti-tippers for the maneuver.
- Position yourself behind the wheelchair rider and place your hands on the push handles. Try not to influence the balance of the wheelchair but be ready to assist the rider if necessary.
- Prevent the wheelchair from tipping backward.
- Keep one hand near the rider's shoulder to prevent a forward fall if the wheelchair comes to an abrupt stop against the curb.
- Provide side-to-side support if the wheelchair begins to tip to one side.
- After completing the maneuver assist with reinstalling or repositioning the anti-tippers.

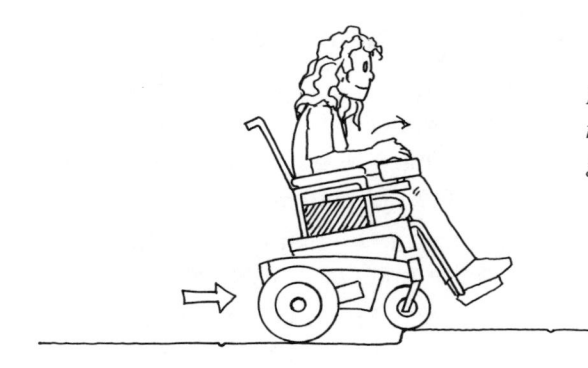

Low curbs and steps may not present a problem going forward.

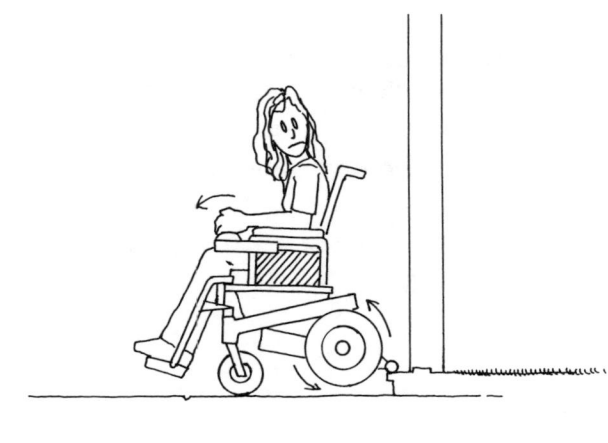

Be aware that your anti-tippers can get caught going down a threshold or a curb.

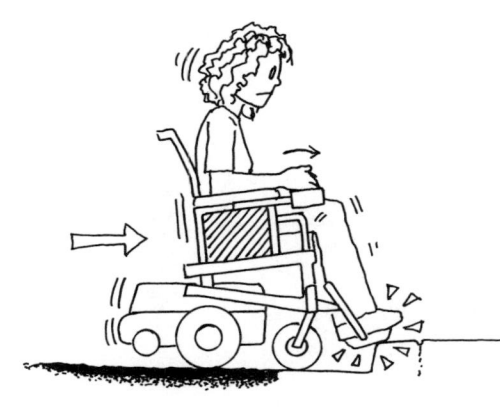

Sometimes the position of your foot supports will prevent you from going up or down a curb easily.

Going up curbs backward independently

Another way to climb curbs is by driving backward. You may not be able to do this if your chair has small anti-tippers in place. Ask your spotter to stand to the side of the wheelchair and be ready to prevent you from falling forward out of your wheelchair.

- Check your anti-tipper clearance. If necessary, have your spotter remove or reposition the anti-tippers for the maneuver.
- Check your foot support clearance. The chair may not be able to tip forward enough to climb a curb driving backward.
- Slowly approach the curb backward until both rear wheels are touching the curb.
- Use your other arm to hold your upper body back in the chair. Drive the wheelchair backward until your rear wheels are on the curb.
- Continue driving backward until the front wheels are on the curb.
- When you have completed the maneuver, have your spotter reinstall or reposition the anti-tippers.

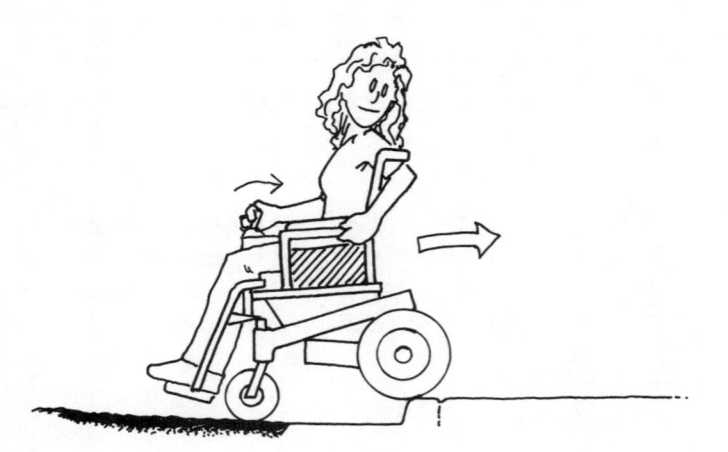

Continue driving backward until the front casters are on the curb.

Going up curbs forward with assistance

If the curb is too high for you to climb independently ask for assistance. The amount of assistance you need will vary depending on the height of the curb.

With one assistant

- Check your anti-tipper clearance. If necessary, have your assistant remove or reposition the anti-tippers for the maneuver.
- Be sure your assistant uses safe body mechanics when pushing by keeping a straight back and by using leg power to push.
- Drive forward until the rear wheels are on the curb.
- If necessary, have your assistant lean into your chair with his or her body weight and push forward and up on the push handles.
- When you have completed the maneuver, have your assistant reinstall or reposition the anti-tippers.

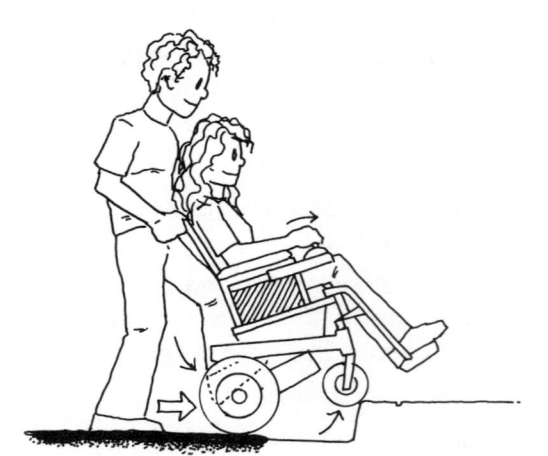

Your assistant can push down and back to help lift the casters onto the curb.

Section 3.7: Curbs and Steps

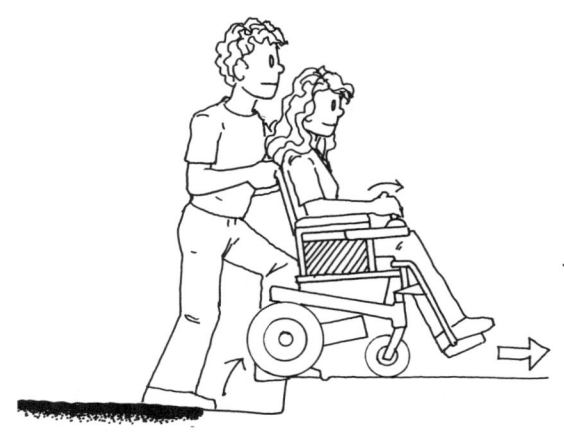

Your assistant may need to push the chair forward from behind until the rear wheels are on the curb.

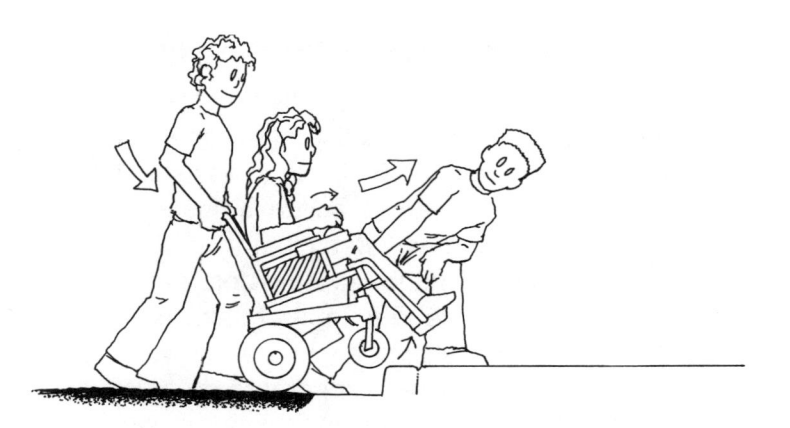

If you need assistance to get up on the curb, have your primary assistant push from behind while a second assistant pulls from the wheelchair frame.

With two assistants

- Check your anti-tipper clearance. If necessary, have an assistant remove or reposition the anti-tippers for the maneuver.
- Drive toward the curb until your foot pedals or front casters are resting against it.
- Ask one assistant to stand to one side of your wheelchair, and bending at the knees, grasp the frame of the wheelchair behind your knees. Be sure the assistant grasps a structural part of the wheelchair and does not hold on to any removable parts.
- The primary assistant should assist from the rear by leaning into your chair with his or her body weight and push forward and up on the push handles.
- On your count of three, have the assistant on the side lift the front of your wheelchair while you slowly drive your wheelchair forward. The assistant(s) only needs to lift the front end high enough so the casters can drive up onto the curb.
- Continue to drive the wheelchair forward until your rear wheels are up on the curb.
- When you have completed the maneuver, have your assistants reinstall or reposition the anti-tippers.

Going Down Curbs

In the presence of a spotter, go down increasingly higher curbs to determine the maximum curb height you can go down independently. Your foot support clearance height and your forward trunk stability will influence the maximum curb height you can go down independently. When backing down curbs, your foot supports may occasionally get caught on the curb. However, you can usually just pull the foot supports off the curb using the power of the motors to back up. If it is a low curb and you are able, it is easier and safer to go forward so you can see where you are going. It is possible to descend small curbs (up to 1 or 2 inches in height), depending on your foot support clearance, by driving forward, but higher curbs might cause you and/or your wheelchair to tip forward. Higher curbs are usually safer to go down backward with assistance. Another consideration when going down curbs in your wheelchair is the clearance underneath the chair. Depending on your wheelbase, backing off a curb that is higher than your ground clearance could result in you getting stuck halfway.

Going down curbs forward independently

While you can descend small curbs slowly, you may find the ride smoother at moderate or full speed. Practice this maneuver in a controlled environment with a spotter available to assist in the event of loss of balance in the forward direction. If descending a curb traveling forward, you must have good clearance under your foot supports. If the foot supports hit the ground before your casters, the wheelchair could come to an abrupt stop. This could throw you forward out of the wheelchair if you are not wearing a lap belt. This could also cause the foot supports to break off. It is also possible that your wheelchair could flip forward on top of you. For this reason, always try to have an assistant present to help when you are practicing, in case of a mishap.

- Check your anti-tipper clearance. If necessary, remove or reposition the anti-tippers for the maneuver.
- Start with very small curbs.
- Facing the curb, drive forward at a moderate speed.
- Shift your weight all the way back (see Section 2.2) and drive the wheelchair perpendicular to the curb or step. Drive forward off of the curb. Be sure both of your front casters leave the curb at the same time to avoid one caster landing before the other.
- Continue driving forward until the rear wheels are off the curb. Ideally, the rear wheels should land just after the front wheels.
- Driving off of a curb at an angle will allow one drive wheel to go down first, causing you to tip over sideways.
- When you have completed the maneuver, reinstall or reposition the anti-tippers.

How a spotter can help

- Check the anti-tipper clearance. If necessary, remove or reposition the anti-tippers for the maneuver.
- Position yourself to the side of the wheelchair.
- You are in a position to prevent the wheelchair rider's upper body from falling forward.
- When you have completed the maneuver, assist with the reinstallation or repositioning of the anti-tippers.

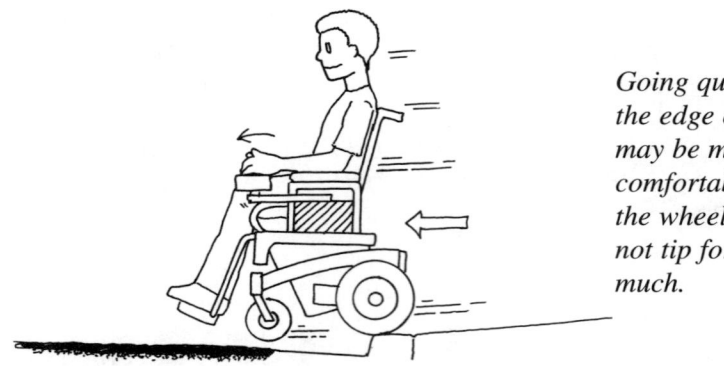

Going quickly over the edge of a curb may be more comfortable because the wheelchair may not tip forward as much.

Going down curbs backward independently

When learning to descend a curb backward, always have a spotter behind your wheelchair to prevent you from tipping over backward.

- Check your anti-tipper clearance. If necessary, remove or reposition the anti-tippers for the maneuver.
- Slowly drive backward until your rear wheels are on the edge of the curb/step.
- Lean forward as far as you can and drive the wheelchair backward until your rear wheels are down.
- Continue to back up until your casters are off the curb/step.
- If your foot supports get caught on the curb/step you may be able to continue driving backward to pull them off.
- When you have completed the maneuver, reinstall or reposition the anti-tippers.

Section 3.7: Curbs and Steps

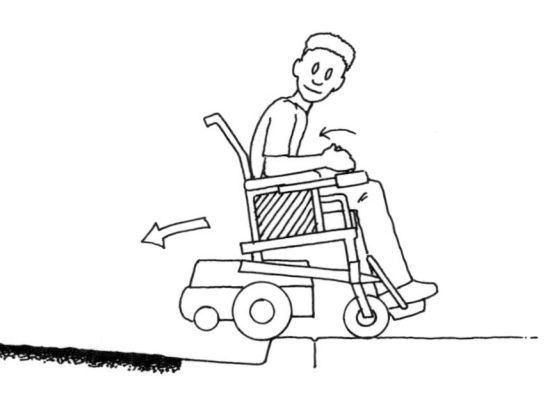

If you do not feel comfortable going down a curb forward, try it backward.

WARNING!

If the height of the curb exceeds your balance point, you could fall over backward performing this maneuver. It is recommended that you always use a spotter behind you when performing this maneuver.

Going down curbs backward with assistance

- Check your anti-tipper clearance. If necessary, have your assistant remove or reposition the anti-tippers for the maneuver.
- Ask your assistant to stand behind you, off the curb or step, with his or her hands on the push handles
- Slowly drive backward until your rear wheels are on the edge of the curb.
- Slowly drive the wheelchair backward until your rear wheels are on the surface below the curb. Your assistant can help slow your descent and control the position of your wheelchair by leaning into the back of your wheelchair using the push handles.
- Continue driving backward until the front casters are on the surface below the curb. Your assistant will need to slowly move backward with you.
- When you have completed the maneuver, have your assistant reinstall or reposition the anti-tippers.

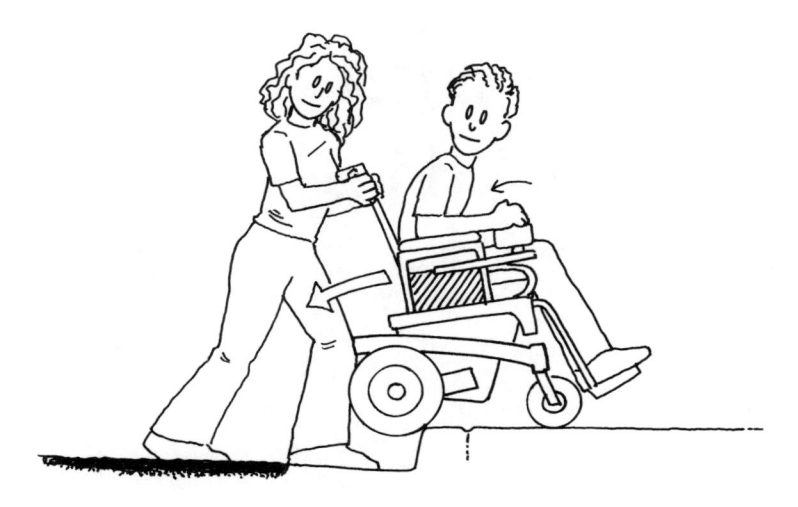

Your assistant can keep your wheelchair from dropping down a curb or step too quickly by "leaning into it" as you slowly back the rear wheels down the curb.

Section 3.8

Elevators and Platform Lifts

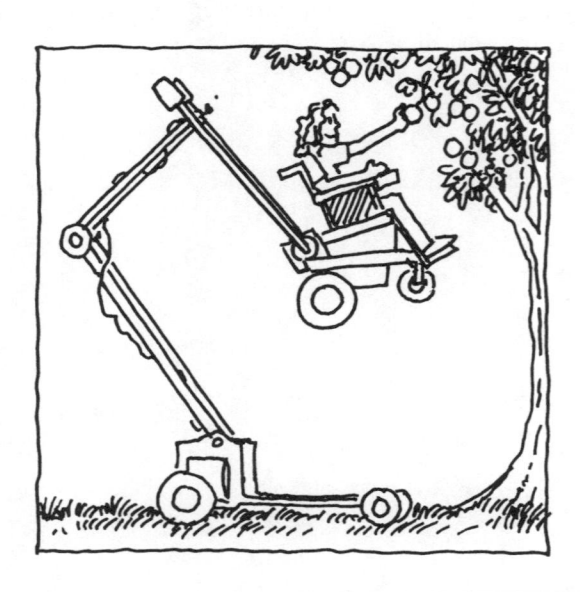

The Americans with Disabilities Act (ADA) imposes strict guidelines that specify how elevators should be constructed to provide access to people with disabilities. These guidelines state that elevator doors should have a minimum width of 36 inches and remain open for at least 5 seconds. See Appendix A for information about the ADA.

Catching an Elevator

Elevator banks

An "elevator bank" is a row of several elevators and is commonly found in places such as hotels and large office buildings. When a person presses the call button, the next available elevator will respond. Though this arrangement sounds convenient, you may find that if the elevator farthest from you opens, you do not have enough time to get on before the doors close. To avoid this problem:

- Position yourself in the center of the elevator bank so you are close to all of the elevators.
- Watch the floor indicators near or above each elevator. When that number nears the number of the floor that you are on, position yourself to catch that elevator.
- Try asking someone to hold the elevator for you.
- Keep pressing the call button until a closer elevator arrives.

If the elevator doors do not remain open for at least 5 seconds, ask the building manager to adjust the timing.

If all the elevators going your direction are full, take one going in the opposite direction and ride it until it changes directions. This often happens if you are on a low floor such as two or three and want to go to the first floor. If the building has many floors, the elevator can be full by the time it reaches you. You can try to wait for another, but if they are continuously full, you will have to do something else. Take one going up and you will be the first one on the elevator as it fills up going back down. Another alternative is to find out where the staff elevators are and use those.

Reaching elevator buttons

Sometimes the floor buttons inside the elevator and the call buttons outside the elevator are out of your reach. They may be too high or could be blocked by a plant or ashtray. To push the button, use a long object, such as a pen, pencil, reacher, flashlight or other handy object. If you do not have anything to push the button with, ask someone for help or try to move the object out of the way using your wheelchair as a plow. Mention the access problem to the building's management and suggest that they move the obstacle. In some elevators, you might have to push the buttons when you are only partway through the door.

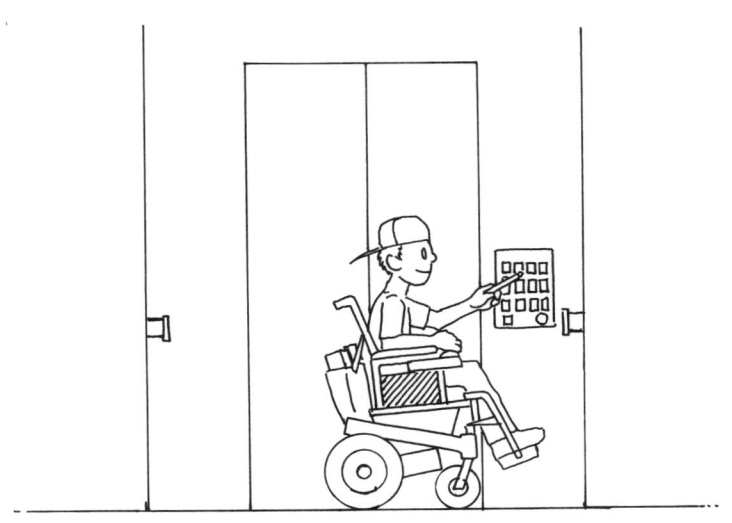

Sometimes you may need to use a pencil or a reacher to press elevator buttons.

Negotiating elevator-to-floor gaps

Elevators are supposed to stop within half an inch of the floor. If there is a vertical or horizontal gap less than 2 inches between the floor and the elevator, negotiate the gap as you would a threshold or curb (see Section 3.2 and 3.7 for more information about thresholds and curbs). If the gap is larger than 2 inches, wait for another elevator rather than risk a hazardous entry.

Negotiating a rise facing forward

- Approach the rise forward.
- Drive forward to get your front wheels up onto the rise. You may need to lean back to reduce the weight on the front casters.
- Without losing momentum, lean forward and keep driving forward until your rear wheels climb up onto the rise.

Negotiating a rise facing backward

- Approach the rise backward.
- Shift your weight back (see Section 2.2) and drive your rear wheels up onto the rise.
- Without losing momentum, keep moving backward until your front wheels move up onto the rise.
- Be sure to watch for people or obstacles that may be behind you.

Negotiating a drop facing forward

- Shift your weight back (see Section 2.2) and drive forward until your front wheels drop to the lower surface.
- Continue moving forward until your rear wheels drop to the lower surface.

Negotiating a drop facing backward

- Lean forward and slowly drive backward until your rear wheels drop to the lower surface.
- Continue moving backward until your front wheels drop to the lower surface.

These techniques are the same for going up and down curbs, which you can review in Section 3.7.

Chapter Three: Navigational Skills

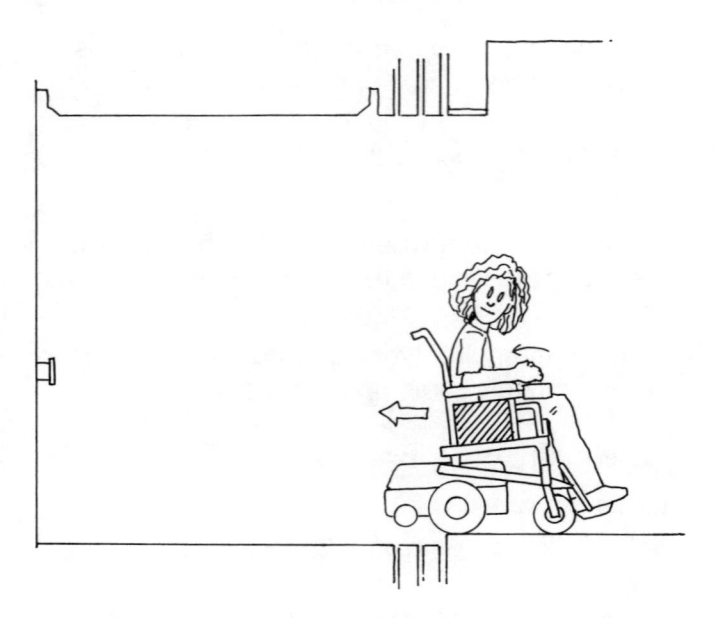

Watch for height differences between the elevator and floor level when you enter and exit elevators.

Entering and Exiting an Elevator

If the elevator is unoccupied and large enough, you may find it easiest to drive in forward and turn around. Then when the elevator reaches your floor, you can drive straight out. If someone will hold the door, you may find it easier to back into the elevator, then you will be in the forward facing position to drive out.

Uncrowded elevators – entering forward

- Enter the elevator facing forward, looking for rises or drops to the elevator floor.
- Turn around inside the elevator to face the door.
- Exit the elevator facing forward, watching for other people, rises or drops to the outside floor level, or other obstacles.

Uncrowded elevators – entering backward

There is more room to maneuver outside the elevator than inside.

- If you are riding the elevator with someone, ask them to hold the door so you can back into the elevator from outside.
- Back into the elevator watching for rises or drops to the elevator floor.
- Exit the elevator facing forward, watching for other people, rises or drops to the outside floor level, and other obstacles.

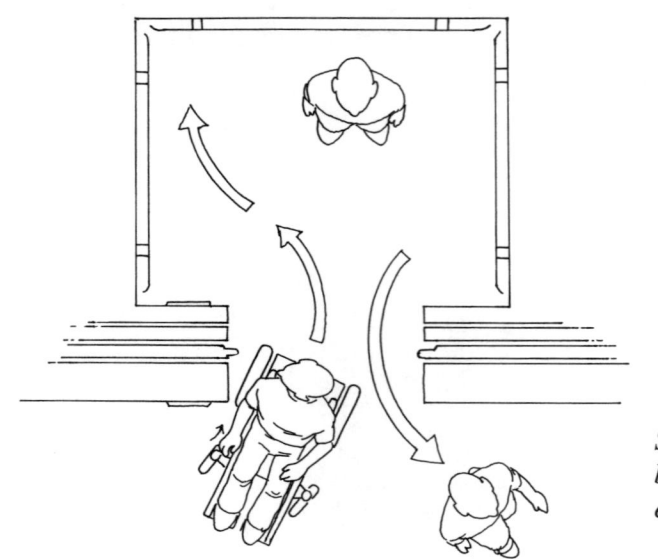

Sometimes backing into an elevator is easiest.

82

Section 3.8: Elevators and Platform Lifts

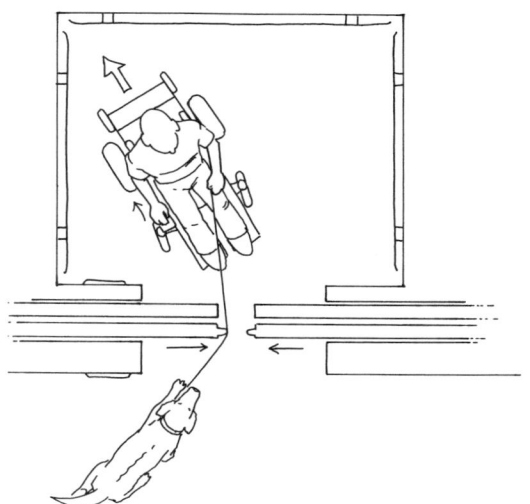

If accompanied by a service dog, don't let it get trapped outside or inside the elevator without you.

Avoid crowded elevators whenever possible.

WARNING!
If you are with a canine companion, be sure that the dog does not end up on one side of the elevator doors while you are on the other. This is especially important if the dog is on a leash! Failure to do so could injure you and your dog.

Crowded elevators

It is usually easier to enter a crowded elevator facing forward. You will be able to see where you are going and others can avoid your foot supports and lean over the front of your chair. It can be difficult for people to get out of the way if you back in.

- Enter the elevator facing forward, watching for a difference in the height of the elevator floor.
- Stay in this position until you reach your floor.
- Exit the elevator facing backward. Be sure to look behind you for other people, rises or drops to the outside floor level, and obstacles.

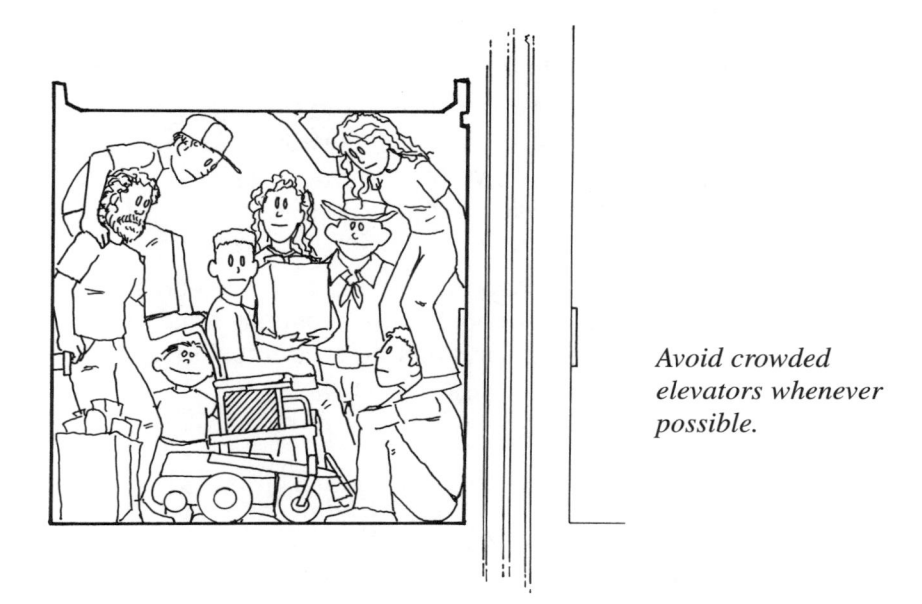

Emergency communication systems

Most elevators have an emergency communication system. Use this phone or other device to summon help in an emergency. Be familiar with the emergency communication system in elevators you use on a regular basis. If you find a problem with the system, notify the management immediately to initiate repairs. Some common problems include:

- The door to the box is difficult to open.
- The communication device is missing or out of order.
- The cord is too short (it should be at least 29 inches long).
- The unit is out of your reach.

Out of service elevators

- Find the front desk or main office. You may also be able to find a "courtesy phone" or borrow a phone (in an apartment, an office, a hotel room, etc.) to call the front desk or main office. They may be able to direct you to an alternative elevator, such as a freight elevator or one specified for employees.

Chapter Three: Navigational Skills

- If necessary, use a phone on the ground floor to call the office you are trying to reach to arrange an alternate meeting site.
- If you are on a high floor in a building and trying to get out, there may be a stair descending track system that can carry you and your wheelchair down the stairway. You will need to locate someone in the building that is familiar with how to operate such an evacuation mechanism.
- If you are riding mass transportation and the only elevator at the transit stop is out of service, you are usually entitled to ride to an alternate station and then to take a taxi to your destination at the transit company's expense.

Platform Lifts

Some buildings have platform lifts instead of ramps or elevators to carry wheelchair riders to another level. The metal platform functions much like the lift on a van. Sometimes these lifts are locked and you will have to find someone with the key. In a public building, the lift should always be left on so you do not have to find the key.

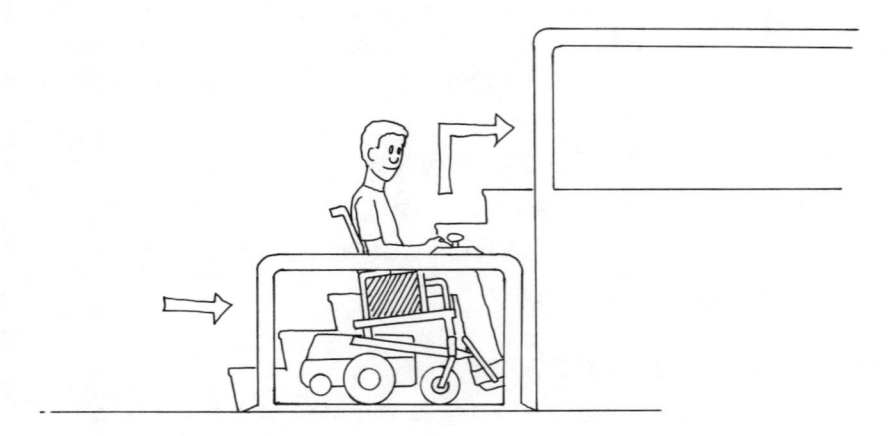

Always try to enter and exit platform lifts facing forward.

Riding on platform lifts

When learning to ride on platform lifts, practice with a spotter nearby. Ask your spotter to make sure all four of your tires are on the platform before you move the lift. Always try to enter and exit platform lifts facing forward. Most platform lifts are constructed so you can roll forward to enter and can continue rolling forward to exit. If the lift requires you to use the same door to both enter and exit, consider backing onto the lift. This way, you can roll forward when exiting.

- Drive onto the lift, making sure all four of your tires are on the platform.
- Set your brakes or lock your wheels.
- Press the button to raise or lower the lift.
- Wait until the lift has come to a complete stop at the top or bottom before releasing your brakes or wheel locks.
- Exit the lift.

How a spotter can help

- Stand in a position that enables you to make sure that all four of the wheelchair tires are on the lift.
- Help operate the lift if necessary.
- Help with the doors on the lift by meeting the wheelchair rider at the top or bottom.

Section 3.9

Tracks and Grates

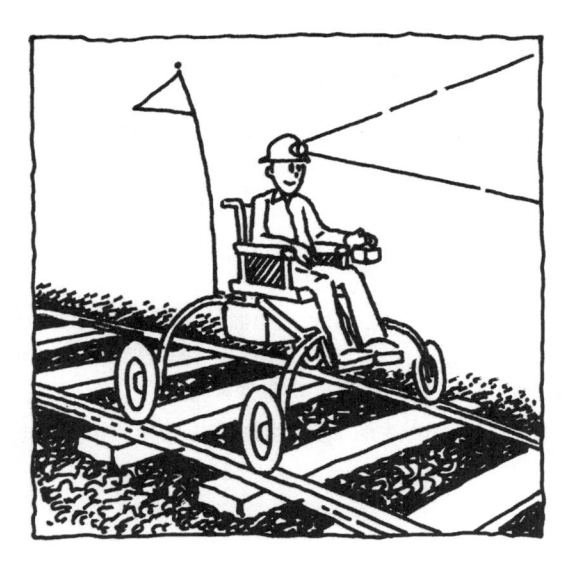

Always examine tracks and grates before you cross them. For tracks, determine how far the rails protrude above or below the traveling surface, and estimate the width of the channels between the rails and traveling surface. For grates, decide whether the drainage slots are wider than your wheels. It is easy to get your casters stuck in these gaps, so be sure to cross perpendicular to the tracks or grate bars. If you cross on four wheels and your casters swivel sideways, they may get stuck in the gaps.

Have a spotter nearby to help you when crossing railroad and trolley tracks so you do not get stuck halfway across. Having a spotter is especially important when crossing tracks unfamiliar to you.

Before practicing the techniques in this section, you should be able to drive a wheelchair forward and backward and cross door thresholds and other obstacles.

Crossing Railroad and Trolley Tracks

- Look at the track and determine if you can cross safely. Do not cross the track if you have any doubts about your safety and make sure someone is available to help if you get stuck.
- Position your wheelchair so that you will cross perpendicular to the tracks.
- Slowly drive forward across the tracks without changing direction.
- Do not deviate from a path perpendicular to the tracks because any turning motion could cause your casters to fall into the gaps along the tracks (see Section 2.5 for more information about caster management).
- There are often dips in the asphalt on either side of the railroad track, which can be very hazardous. Move slowly to avoid tipping backward.

If you feel the tracks are too high to cross without catching your front wheels, you may want to try and develop a technique to cross them backward. Be sure you can clear your anti-tippers and foot supports before trying to cross tracks.

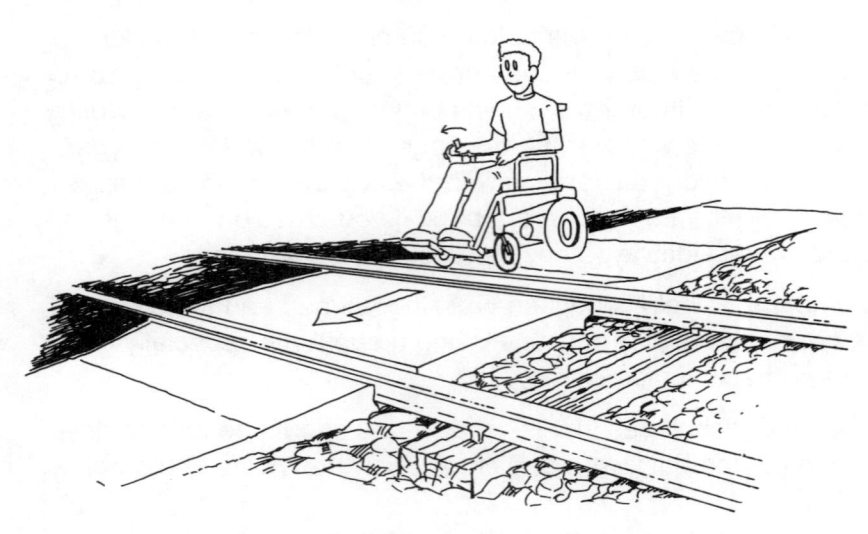

Cross railroad tracks in the forward direction with momentum to avoid getting your casters caught. Your wheelchair should be perpendicular to the tracks when crossing.

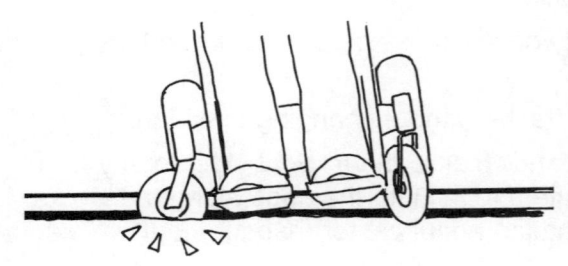

Do not deviate from a path perpendicular to the tracks, because any turning motion could cause your casters to pivot and then drop into the gap next to the track.

WARNING!
Crossing large gaps can be dangerous. Practice with a spotter until you are confident doing this maneuver alone. If you get caught in a train track alone you could get run over by a train!

How a spotter can help
- Walk next to the non-joystick side of the wheelchair rider. Be ready to catch the wheelchair rider at the trunk if the wheels catch and the rider loses upper body balance.
- If the wheelchair gets stuck, move to the back of the chair. Push down and forward on the push handles. On a rear-wheel drive chair, this will raise the front casters and assist in moving the wheelchair forward.

Crossing Grates

Whether you live in the city or the country, you are likely to encounter either sewer grates or cattle guards. Grates are supposed to be positioned so the longer openings are perpendicular to the most common path of travel. Grate openings should not be more than half an inch wide. Since many grates do not meet these standards, it is best to avoid crossing directly over them whenever possible. If you must cross a grate, go slowly and plot a course perpendicular to the grate slots.

Wide slots and a lack of crossbars make cattle guards an extreme version of sewer grates. Like grates, cross cattle guards perpendicular to the bars. However, you might need help from an assistant to keep your casters from turning and dropping into an opening.

With a spotter, practice crossing different grates. You can often find grates on city sidewalks and at the base of driveways and curb ramps.

Basic grate crossing
- Cross perpendicular to the length of the opening in the grate. Do not cross the grate parallel to the length of the openings or the casters may drop into the grate.
- Drive slowly to prevent a sudden stop if the casters drop into the grate.

- Drive forward without turning. Turning slightly may cause the casters to turn and drop into the grate openings.
- The assistant or assistants should lift at the casters of the wheelchair to keep them from turning and dropping down into the grate.

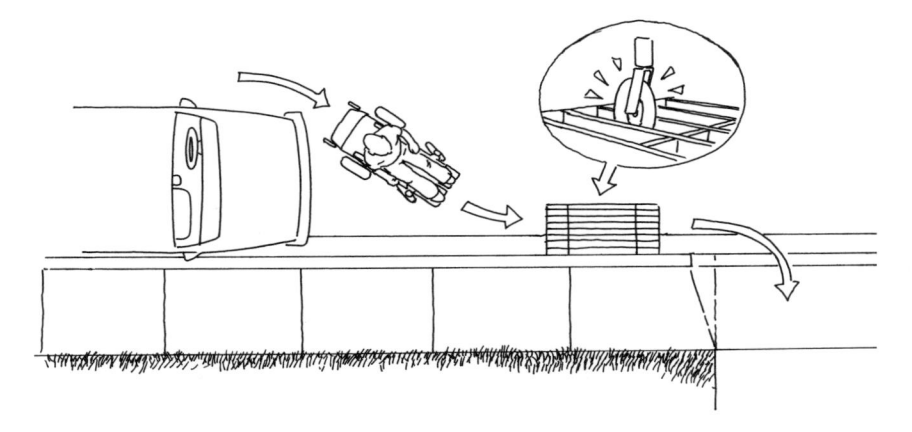

Do not drive parallel to the openings in a grate; your casters may drop into the grate.

If your casters get stuck, try to back off the grate. Be aware that this may be difficult because casters will try to turn from forward to backward when the direction of travel shifts. You will potentially need assistance to lift the casters up and out of the grate.

Grates with longer openings parallel to the path of travel

- If you cross this type of grate by driving straight over it, your wheels can get caught in the grooves of the grate.
- Try crossing the grate openings at an angle.

How a spotter can help

- Walk on the non-joystick side of the wheelchair. Be ready to catch the wheelchair rider if the casters get stuck and the rider loses upper body balance.
- If the casters get stuck in the grate, push down and forward on the push handles to raise the casters and help move the chair forward.
- You can also lift the front of the wheelchair as the rider slowly drives forward, if the casters are stuck in the grate.

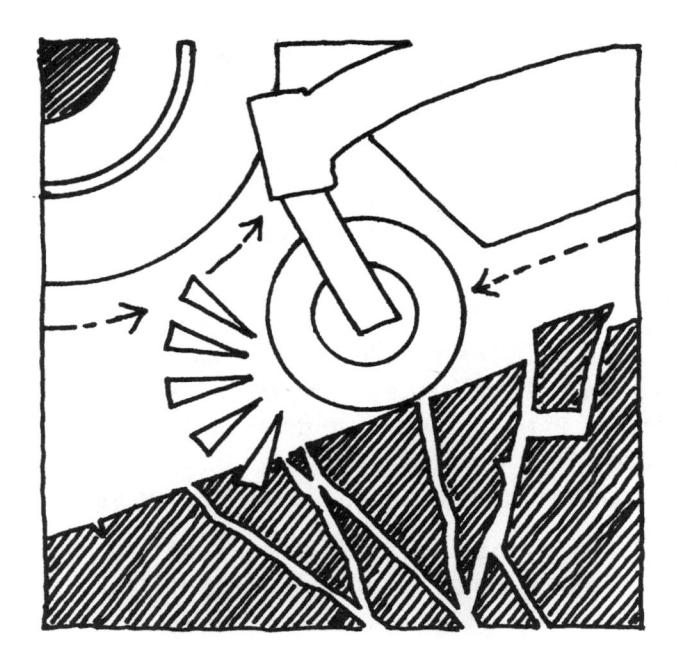

Emergency Skills

CHAPTER 4

In this Chapter

4.1	Stairs	90
4.2	Falling and Getting Up	93
4.3	Electromagnetic Compatibility	97
4.4	Evacuation Procedures	100

Fire! The smoke is rising fast to your floor, and the incandescent glow of flames has reached the floor below you. People are screaming, choking in the smoke, and running down the fire escapes. You rush to the hall – the elevators are dead. What do you do now?

The stress and panic of an emergency can make it difficult to think clearly and act wisely. Practice disaster and safety procedures in advance so that you will be calmer and react appropriately in an actual emergency.

The skills in this chapter may expose you and any assistants helping you to physical strain and serious injury. Read the warnings on page xi to learn about the risks involved in performing wheelchair skills. Falling is an unacceptable option for some wheelchair riders that may result in severe injury or death.

Chapter Four: Emergency Skills

Section 4.1

Stairs

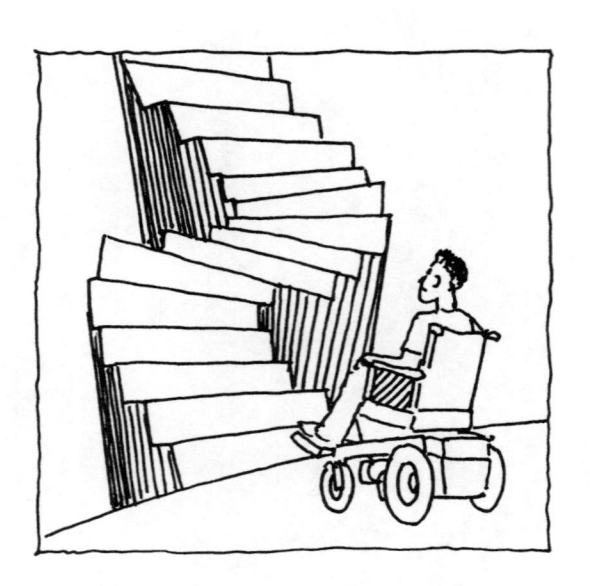

Powered wheelchairs are too heavy to routinely travel up and down stairs with any frequency. This is generally considered an emergency maneuver, unless you really want to get somewhere that you cannot get to by an accessible route. Laying a portable ramp on the stairs is definitely the preferred solution. Even in an emergency, it may be safest to leave your powered wheelchair behind if time is critical to get out of the building. If there are only one or two steps going into a restaurant, and the steps have long landings, you might not mind asking for help.

This chapter deals with flights of stairs. Only negotiate flights of stairs in a powered wheelchair during an emergency. An elevator may be out of service, or it may be temporarily out of order, in need of repair. In most cases, it is easiest and safest to wait until the elevator is repaired. If this is not possible, and there is no other way, you and your assistants will have to negotiate the stairs.

Keep a manual wheelchair at places you frequent, such as work, so that you will have a backup chair to use in emergencies. If such an emergency occurs, exit using the manual wheelchair and leave your powered wheelchair behind.

The techniques in this section can help you ascend and descend stairs in flights, not single steps. Single or very widely spaced steps can be managed using the techniques for curbs described in Section 3.7.

Only perform the techniques in this section if you absolutely must use the stairs in an emergency and there is no other accessible alternative available. These techniques require a significant amount of wheelchair experience and strength to accomplish, and may expose you and any assistants to physical strain and serious injury. Keep in mind that your wheelchair alone may weigh 250 pounds, then add your own weight to that. If you decide to practice these techniques, start with wide, deep stairs equipped with handrails and attempt progressively steeper stairs until you are no longer comfortable. If the steps are too shallow to accommodate your wheels, it may be hazardous to negotiate the stairs. Only practice stair techniques if multiple assistants are present.

Going Up Stairs

How to ask for assistance

Be sure your assistants use proper body mechanics when carrying your wheelchair up the stairs (see Section 6.1 for more information about preventing injuries).

- Ideally, you will want to have at least three able-bodied individuals to assist you and your wheelchair up the stairs.
- If you can be transferred from your wheelchair and can wait at the top or bottom of the stairs, instruct your assistants to assist you in transferring from your wheelchair to another chair.
- Disengage the drive wheels to be able to push the chair.
- Have the assistants turn the wheelchair off and position it to go up the stairs forward.
- One assistant should be positioned at the rear of the wheelchair, with their hands on the push handles. This person's job will be to guide and push the wheelchair up the stairs.
- Have the other two assistants stand on either side of the wheelchair, grasping structural parts of the wheelchair (not a removable part, such as an arm support or leg support). It is their job to help lift and pull the wheelchair up the stairs.
- Have the assistants roll, push, and lift the wheelchair up the steps, one step at a time. On the count of three, they should push, lift and roll up each step, one at a time. Be sure they are keeping their backs straight and are using their legs for strength instead of the weaker arm and back muscles.
- When the wheelchair is safely at the top of the stairs, ask your assistants to carry you up the stairs using the most appropriate technique (see Section 4.2 for some sample techniques).
- Be sure to re-engage the motors to the rear wheels.

If you cannot be transferred from your wheelchair and you are in an emergency situation, follow the same technique as above with you seated in the wheelchair. A fourth person is recommended to assist at the rear to help push and lift up the stairs.

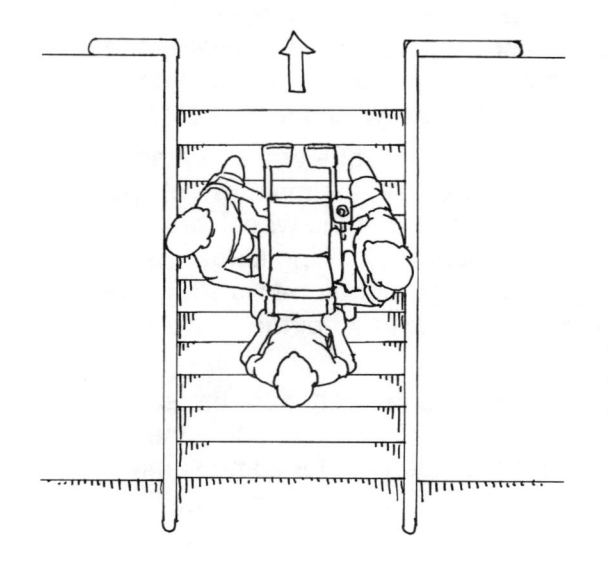

Pushing and lifting a powered wheelchair up stairs requires at least three assistants.

Going Down Stairs

How to ask for assistance

Be sure your assistants use proper body mechanics when carrying your wheelchair down the stairs (see Section 6.1 for more information about preventing injuries).

- Ideally, you will want to have at least three able-bodied individuals to assist you and your wheelchair down the stairs.
- If you can be transferred from your wheelchair and can wait at the top or bottom of the stairs, instruct your assistants to assist you in transferring from your wheelchair to another chair.
- Disengage the drive wheels to be able to push the chair.
- Have the assistants turn the wheelchair off and position it to go down the stairs backward.
- One assistant should lean into the rear of the wheelchair while holding the push handles. This person's job will be to guide the wheelchair as it slowly rolls down, one step at a time.

- Have the other two assistants stand on either side of the wheelchair, grasping structural parts of the wheelchair (not a removable part, such as an arm support or leg support). It is their job to help guide the wheelchair and slow the descent.
- Have the assistants step down the stairs one at a time, rolling the wheelchair slowly as they go. As the main wheels pass each step, the assistant at the rear of the wheelchair can maintain control of the wheelchair by rolling it down onto the next step. Be sure they are keeping their backs straight and are using their legs for strength instead of the weaker arm and back muscles.
- When the wheelchair is safely at the bottom of the stairs, ask your assistants to carry you down the stairs using the most appropriate technique (see Section 4.2 for some sample techniques).
- Be sure to re-engage the motors to the rear wheels.

If you cannot be transferred from your wheelchair and you are in an emergency situation, follow the same technique as above with you seated in the wheelchair. Use extreme caution.

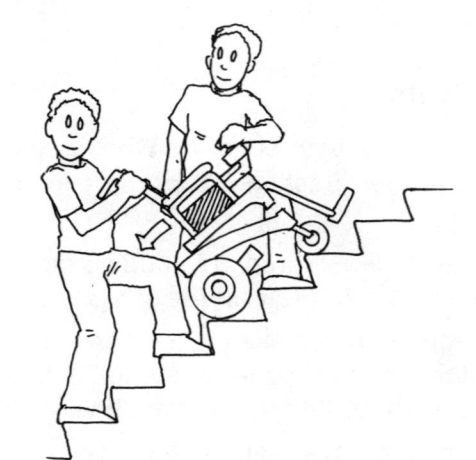

The assistant at the rear should lean into the back of the wheelchair to control the rate of descent.

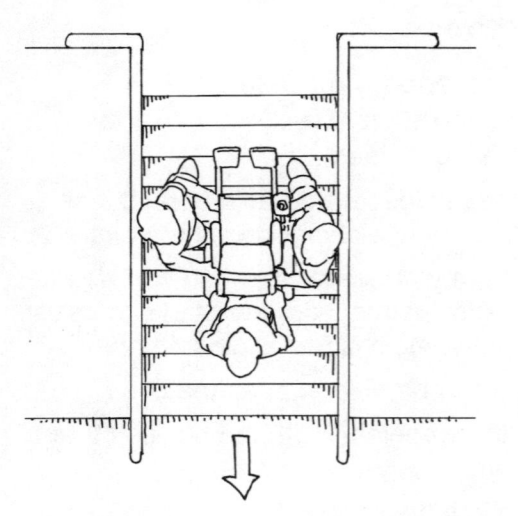

Carrying a powered wheelchair down stairs requires at least three assistants.

Section 4.2

Falling and Getting Up

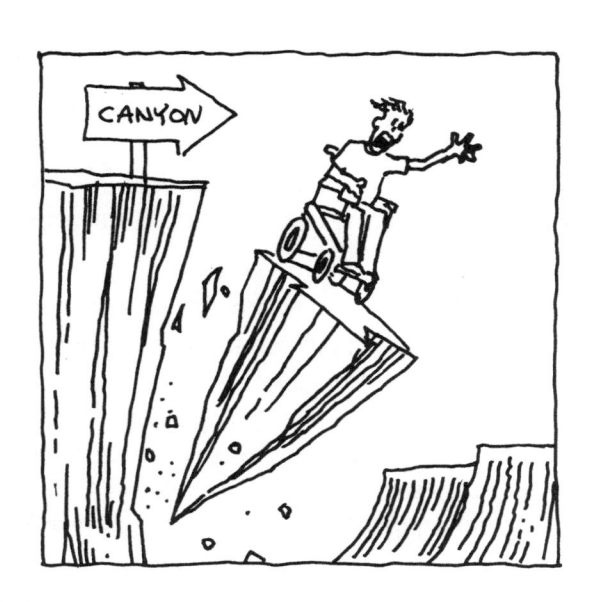

Learning how to fall and get back into your wheelchair are critical safety skills. It is best to learn these skills with the coaching and supervision of a physical or occupational therapist with wheelchair training experience in a rehab environment. You should know how to fall and get up, or be able to instruct others to help you get back into your wheelchair.

Falling

At one time or another, you may tip over in your powered wheelchair. If you opt for a less stable chair setup to gain more maneuverability, you might be more likely to fall. Even if you are careful, the terrain over which you ride could cause your powered wheelchair to tip over. If you do fall, you can act to protect yourself.

Falling backward

- Always protect you head!
- If you start falling backward, tuck your chin into your chest. This will prevent your head from hitting the ground first.
- Hold your knees back with both hands or keep them away from your face with an arm.

Falling forward

- If you do not have a lap belt on, try to curl into a ball so you will roll out of the wheelchair. Putting your arms out in front of you to stop your fall can result in a broken arm or wrist.

Falling sideways

- Lean in the opposite direction of the fall to prevent your head from hitting the ground.
- Place both arms on the arm support in the opposite direction of the fall so the chair hits the ground before you do. Don't catch yourself by reaching out an arm because you could sustain a wrist, elbow or shoulder injury. Do not let your arm get caught underneath the wheelchair as you fall.

Practice fall

Practicing these falling techniques may be helpful for some wheelchair riders in preparing for a fall. However, even under controlled and supervised conditions, falling exposes you and any assistants helping you, to a potentially harmful situation. For some wheelchair riders, falling may result in severe injury or death. If you do practice falling, make sure experienced therapists are present at all times. When simulating a fall, most therapists will tip the chair very slowly until it reaches the ground. This will simulate a fall in slow motion. If you do practice falling, practice on a soft surface like a mat, grass, futon, or soft sand.

How a spotter can help

- Stand behind the wheelchair with your hands on the push handles or on the back posts.
- Turn your body sideways and push your hip into the back of the wheelchair. To avoid back injuries, do not twist at the waist. When the wheelchair rider is ready, tip the chair into a wheelie.
- Slowly lower the wheelchair to the floor.

Battery Acid

Battery acid can burn you if it comes in contact with your skin. When you fall, your chair might also tip and fall over, jarring the batteries. If you use batteries containing battery acid, avoid letting leaked acid touch your skin, and caution any assistants about this as well. Be sure to ask your assistant to move you away from any battery acid that may have spilled. There is no danger of leaking acid from gel cell or sealed acid batteries because the chambers are sealed.

> **WARNING!**
> Lead acid batteries that are not sealed with gelled acid are dangerous. Sealed, maintenance free batteries, like those in your car, do not have gelled acid and can be just as dangerous. Replace your batteries with sealed gel cells.

If you do get into a situation where the battery acid leaks:
- Do not touch the acid.
- If the acid touches your skin or clothes, immediately wash with soap and water.
- If the acid gets into your eyes, immediately flush your eyes with cold running water. Do this for at least 10 minutes and seek medical attention immediately.

Getting Up

It is important for you to know the safest and easiest way to be lifted from the ground to your wheelchair. Your best bet is to instruct others how they can get you back into your wheelchair. This transfer should be taught/learned with the counseling and supervision of therapists in a rehab environment. Not only will this transfer be necessary when you fall, but also in other situations, such as if you go on a picnic and want to sit on your cushion on the ground with your friends.

If you fall, the first thing you will probably have to do is calm down other people around you. Make sure they stop and regroup so you can all work together. If the wheelchair has fallen on top of you, have them move it. It is always a good idea to have someone call Emergency 911, because you may not realize the extent of any injuries. Regardless, you might want to go to the emergency room for a thorough inspection of your body and to have X-rays taken to check for fractures, especially if you have limited or no pain sensation.

Before getting up

- Check for any broken bones or injuries you might have. Be especially careful inspecting areas where you do not have full sensation.
- Make sure the wheelchair is turned off.
- You may want to be sure all your "plumbing" (leg bag, catheter, etc.) is in place.
- Seek medical assistance to verify that you do not have any hidden injuries.
- Finally, check for damage to your wheelchair. Make sure all parts are in their proper position, including your arm supports, back support, and leg supports. Verify that your chair still works.

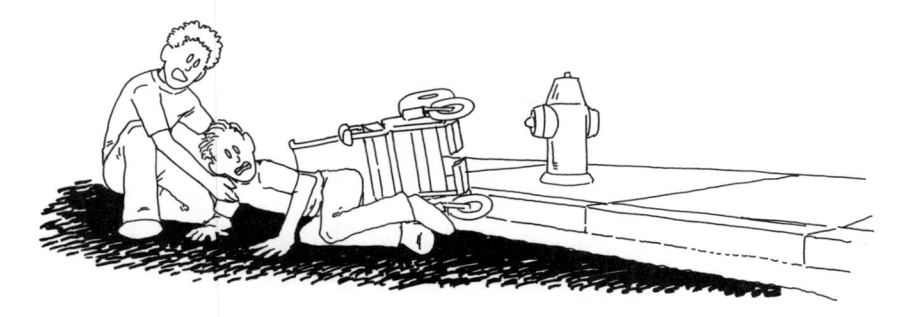

Check for injuries before you get back up.

Getting up from a fall

If the wheelchair has tipped completely over backward and you are still in the wheelchair, a couple of assistants may be able to tip the wheelchair back upright with you in it.

If you have fallen completely out of your wheelchair but the wheelchair is still upright and there is no damage to the wheelchair, transfer from the ground to your wheelchair using the techniques you learned in rehab. This may require you to instruct others on how they can assist you. Practice explaining these procedures to trained therapists to learn the proper verbal instructions for the type of transfer you need.

If you have fallen over to the side, but are still in the wheelchair, it might be possible for a few assistants to tilt the wheelchair back in place with you still in it. However, it may be safer and easier for you to be moved to a safe place while your chair is righted. Next, have your assistants help you back into the chair.

How to ask for assistance

Using an assistant to help is sometimes the quickest, easiest, and most convenient way to get back in your wheelchair. Ask your regular assistant to read Chapter 6 for more information about assisting safely. There are several methods to help you into your wheelchair.

With one assistant – Fireman's carry

- Clasp your hands around your assistant's shoulders.
- Have your assistant cradle you around the back with one arm and grasp you under the knees with the other.
- On your count of three, have your assistant lift straight up. From this position, the assistant can walk to your wheelchair and place you in the seat.
- Make sure your assistant bends at the knees, not the back, when lifting you.

Chapter Four: Emergency Skills

With an assistant at your head and at your feet

- Cross your arms in front of you.
- Have one assistant stand behind you, reaching under your arms to grab your wrists.
- Have the second assistant stand in front of you and reach forward under your legs to support your knees and/or feet.
- On your count of three, both assistants should lift you up and move you over to your wheelchair seat.
- Make sure your assistants bend at the knees and keep their backs as vertical as possible to avoid back injuries.

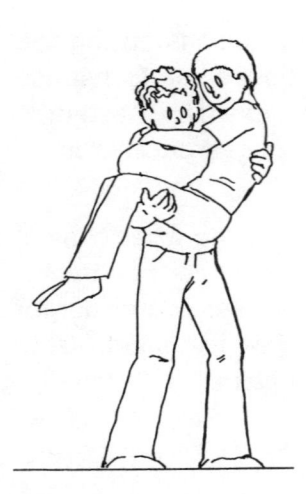

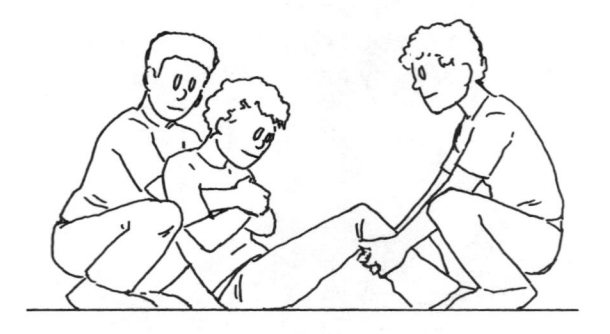

Fireman's carry – If your assistant is strong enough, you can be lifted back into your chair using the fireman's carry.

With an assistant on each side - Wedding seat carry

- Have your assistants stand on either side of you.
- Put an arm behind each person's shoulder as your assistants lock arms around your back and under your knees.
- On your count of three, both assistants should lift you up and move you over into your wheelchair seat.
- Make sure your assistants bend at the knees and keep their backs as vertical as possible to avoid back injuries.

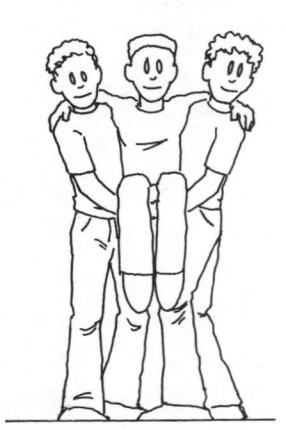

Wedding seat carry – Two assistants can form a seat with their arms to lift you back into your wheelchair.

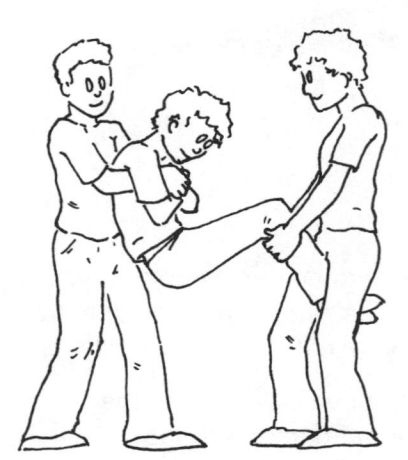

Have one assistant lift you under the arms from behind, clasping your arms across your chest, while the other assistant holds you under the knees.

96

Section 4.3
Electromagnetic Compatibility

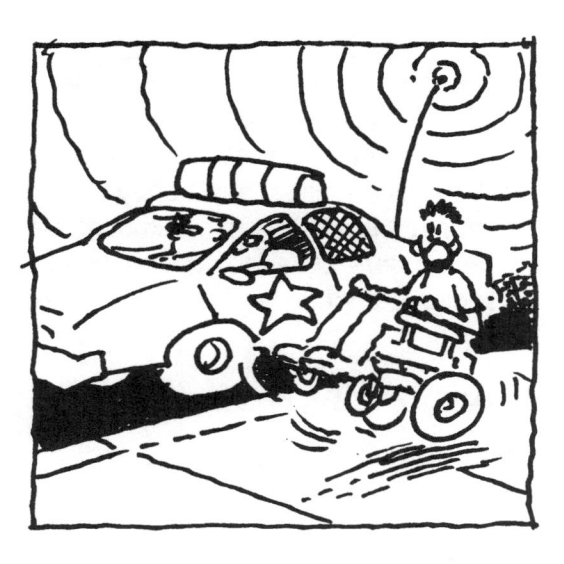

Almost all electronic and electromechanical devices give off some amount of electromagnetic energy. This energy is also called radio frequency emissions. Similarly, electromagnetic energy can affect the operation of almost any electronic or electronically controlled device. Most of the time, the amount or level of electromagnetic energy in a given environment is too low for anything to happen. Sometimes the amount of energy is high enough to affect the operation of a device, resulting in a phenomenon called Electromagnetic Interference (EMI) or Radio Frequency Interference (RFI). For example, if a vacuum cleaner is operated very close to a television set, you might see "snow" on the television screen.

For your powered wheelchair, the response to high levels of electromagnetic energy could be dangerous. The wheelchair may stop, the chair may move erratically or veer off in one direction or another while you are in motion, or the brakes may release, causing the chair to start moving. For these reasons, powered wheelchairs should be designed to be resistant to electromagnetic energy. Some wheelchair models are more resistant to electromagnetic energy than others, and not all wheelchairs have been tested to verify their resistance. However, even if tested, a strong enough level of electromagnetic energy could cause problems for any powered wheelchair.

Other potential electromagnetic compatibility problems related to powered wheelchairs stem from radio frequency emissions from your own wheelchair affecting other electronic or electromechanical devices that you might be using on or near your wheelchair. This type of interference is more likely to occur when the wheelchair is being driven than when the wheelchair is stopped. It can also be more likely when the wheelchair batteries are being charged. Ideally, a cell phone, amateur (HAM) radio, laptop computer, breathing machine, or other device that you might also use will be designed to resist such interference. Some models of these types of devices will be more resistant to this energy than others, and those that have been tested to meet appropriate electromagnetic compatibility (EMC) standards are more likely to operate properly than models that have not been tested.

Electrostatic discharge, or "static electricity," is another potential problem that could affect your chair's performance. If you have ever experienced a slight electrical shock or spark when touching someone or something else, you have experienced electrostatic discharge. When any portion of your wheelchair comes close to touching something with a different electrical charge, it can experience the same sort of electrical shock. Depending on the strength and location of this shock, it could cause an undesired response by your wheelchair.

Charging your wheelchair batteries also creates a potential situation for an EMI event. The cable from your charger to your wheelchair is a potential pathway for electromagnetic energy to find its way into your wheelchair. Wheelchairs that meet recognized EMC standards have circuits that prevent driving while charging; however, it is always a good practice to turn your wheelchair off while you are charging it.

Sources of Electromagnetic Energy

The most common sources of electromagnetic energy that may cause problems for your powered wheelchair are usually completely separate from your wheelchair, such as radio and TV transmitters. Your chair's ability to resist interference depends on:

- The frequency and amount of power transmitted by the source
- The distance you are from the transmitter
- The presence of other metallic objects around you that might either reflect energy toward, or deflect energy away from, your wheelchair
- The design of your wheelchair

For example, a police radio transmitter on a patrol car will put out more energy than a hand held radio. However, if the hand held radio is very close to you while it is transmitting, your wheelchair could experience a higher level of electromagnetic energy from the hand held transmitter than from the police radio transmitter.

Problems caused by EMI events may occur when the radio waves in the vicinity of a powered wheelchair are stronger than the wheelchair was designed to resist. The strength of radio waves is measured in units of volts per meter (V/m). Strong sources of electromagnetic energy that may cause EMI to occur include, but are not limited to:

- Cellular phones
- Amateur (HAM) radios
- Citizens band (CB) radios
- Radio station transmitters
- Television station transmitters
- Two-way radios used by police, fire fighters, and ambulances
- Two-way radios used by taxi cabs
- Two-way radios used by aircraft
- "Walkie-talkies" used by security guards, factory employees, or surveyors
- High power electrical installations (e.g. power transformers, electric railways or tramways)
- Lightning
- Medical equipment such as CAT scanners or X-ray machines
- Radar transmitters
- Aircraft

Many commonly used radio transmitters typically radiate too little power to cause EMI. These low power transmitters include garage door openers, keyless entry devices for vehicles, cordless telephones, children's walkie-talkies, and hobby radio controls for model boats or airplanes. While it is not impossible for these types of radio transmitters to cause an EMI event, it is much less likely to occur because they do not transmit with much power.

Dealing with EMI

EMI events occur now and will continue to occur in the future. The degree of protection a wheelchair has against EMI is known as its level of immunity. The Food and Drug Administration (FDA) currently recommends that powered wheelchairs should be designed with a level of immunity of at least 20 volts per meter. Some of the powered wheelchairs that are currently on the market do not meet this minimum recommendation, and are much more likely to experience EMI events than wheelchairs that do. Conversely, some wheelchairs provide greater protection than the FDA minimum recommendation.

All new wheelchairs are now required to have a label disclosing the level of immunity to which the wheelchair has been tested. Wheelchairs that have labels showing a higher level of immunity provide a greater degree of protection. The FDA also allows wheelchair manufacturers to market wheelchairs that are labeled "Not Tested." These wheelchairs typically will not meet the FDA minimum immunity recommendation.

Before you start losing too much sleep, remember that experiencing an EMI event in a powered wheelchair is rare.

Reducing the risks during an EMI event

- If your wheelchair starts to move on its own, you will want to turn off the power immediately.
- Practice turning off your wheelchair. This way, if you suddenly lose control of your wheelchair due to an EMI event (or any other reason), you will be familiar with the procedure for turning off the power to stop the wheelchair.
- While you are driving slowly, practice turning off your wheelchair with a spotter available to assist if necessary.
- Be prepared for a sudden stop, which may pitch you forward.
- Be cautious when you turn the wheelchair back on. If the source of the EMI event is a mobile transmitter that has driven away, you will be able to continue driving normally when the source of electromagnetic energy is no longer present.

- Unless the wheelchair manufacturer specifies otherwise, always turn your wheelchair off in the presence of a radio transmitter such as a cellular phone or CB radio.
- Leave your wheelchair turned off when you are parked.

Cellular phones

A cellular phone can be a tremendous asset for a powered wheelchair user. If the manufacturer does not specify the compatibility of your wheelchair with a cell phone, your safest bet is to turn your wheelchair off before answering your cell phone.

If you plan to use a cellular phone, it is important to determine the compatibility of your phone with your wheelchair while both are in use.

- Be extremely cautious.
- Have a spotter with you who is instructed to immediately turn off the power on your wheelchair if there is any problem.
- Put your cellular phone through a number of tests by using it to make several calls and determine if there is a compatibility problem that causes your wheelchair to operate in any erratic or unexpected manner.
- Make sure that you will not be so distracted by using your cellular phone that it adversely affects your ability to safely operate your wheelchair.

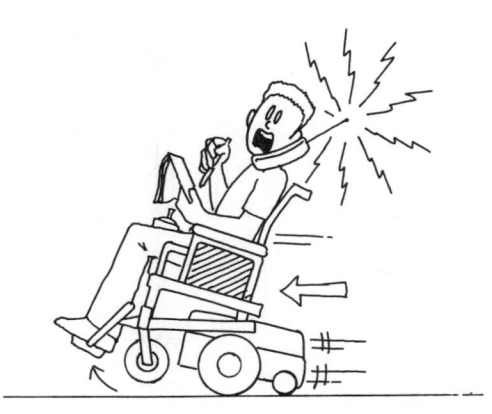

Using a cell phone near your wheelchair while it is turned on could cause an EMI event and make your wheelchair operate erratically.

Section 4.4

Evacuation Procedures

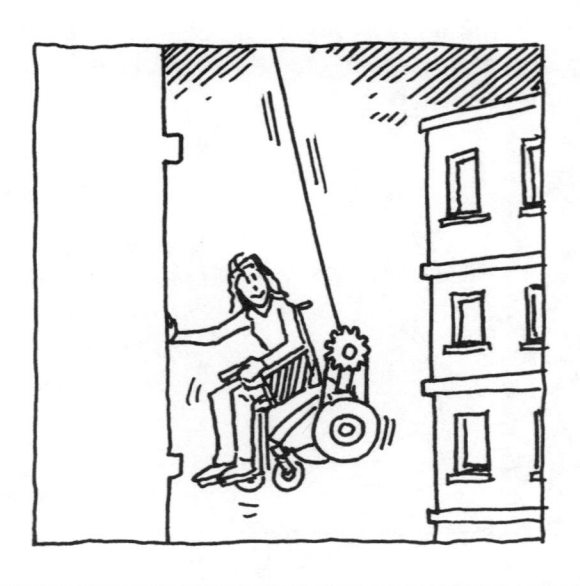

It is a good idea to have an emergency evacuation plan for your home, workplace, school, or other places where you spend a lot of time. Make sure your smoke detectors are working and that you can reach a fire extinguisher and fire alarm pull. Find out if there is a safety plan at your apartment building, school or worksite. Know what to do and where to go during each emergency situation (e.g. earthquake, tornado, fire). Know the evacuation route at your home, school and work place. Have an alternate route planned as well.

A formal evacuation plan for wheelchair riders that does not require the use of an elevator should be established for buildings with more than one story. Learn the recommended evacuation plan. In some places, this might mean using an evacuation track device, which attaches to a wheelchair and enables it to negotiate stairs with assistance. If an adaptive evacuation device is not available, consider asking a coworker or friend to carry you out, leaving the wheelchair behind. Relying on other people can be dangerous because they may not always be available.

If you spend a significant amount of time on an upper floor of a building with an elevator, check with the building management and the fire department to verify if you will be able to use the elevator as the safest exit method if it is determined that the fire is not in that sector.

Perhaps the safest alternative is to have your home or work place on the ground floor so that evacuation is possible. A second floor could be ramped for evacuation purposes as well.

Designate assistants (e.g. family members, roommates, coworkers, classmates, teachers) who will help you in an emergency. Practice the evacuation with your assistants. Be sure they know how to maneuver your wheelchair if you are unable to do so yourself, as well as how to carry you safely if you cannot evacuate in your wheelchair. Your assistants can use a blanket or curtain as a cradle to carry you down flights of stairs if necessary.

You will probably spend a lot of time out of your wheelchair at home. Teach family members, attendants, friends, and/or roommates how to get you in and out of the wheelchair for a quick evacuation. Designate a meeting area outside your home. Be sure your neighbors know you use a wheelchair. This information is helpful for rescuers.

Local police and fire departments should be equipped with a floor plan of the home and the typical sleeping location of individuals with severe disabilities. In the event of a fire or emergency evacuation, emergency personnel will know where to find and assist individuals unable to self-evacuate.

Creating an Emergency Plan

- Designate emergency contacts and keep their phone numbers available. If you are separated from your family, use this number as an "emergency headquarters."
- Keep a first aid kit available. You may want to include information about your medical condition and a list of your physician(s), as well as medication(s), a tire pump, a flashlight, and other medical supplies.
- Take courses in first aid, CPR and self-defense.
- Carry a cell phone in case you need to call for help.

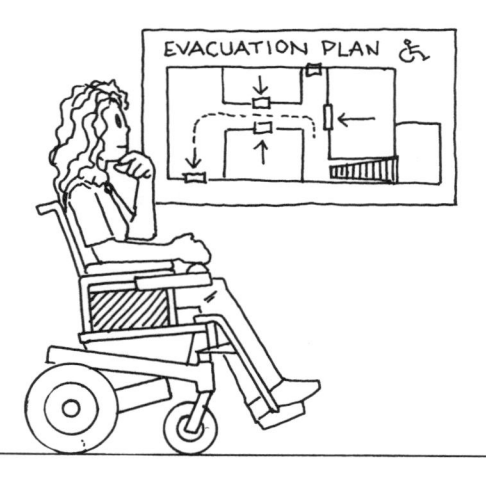

Evacuation plans should be available at work, schools, recreation facilities and even at home.

Personal Emergency

Make sure others know about your personal medical condition. If you have a spinal cord injury and are susceptible to conditions such as autonomic dysreflexia, be sure that family members are aware of the symptoms and what to do if you have them. Keep your treatment information available in case you have a medical emergency. Train those around you in emergency care techniques such as elevating your feet if your blood pressure drops or transferring you to the floor for emergency rescue purposes. Do not be afraid to call 911.

If you have a personal emergency and need to be taken to a hospital, emergency medical personnel find the following helpful:

- A list of current medications and dosages
- A current supply of medications in a labeled container from a pharmacy
- A Medic Alert bracelet listing allergies, specific conditions, and/or medications required

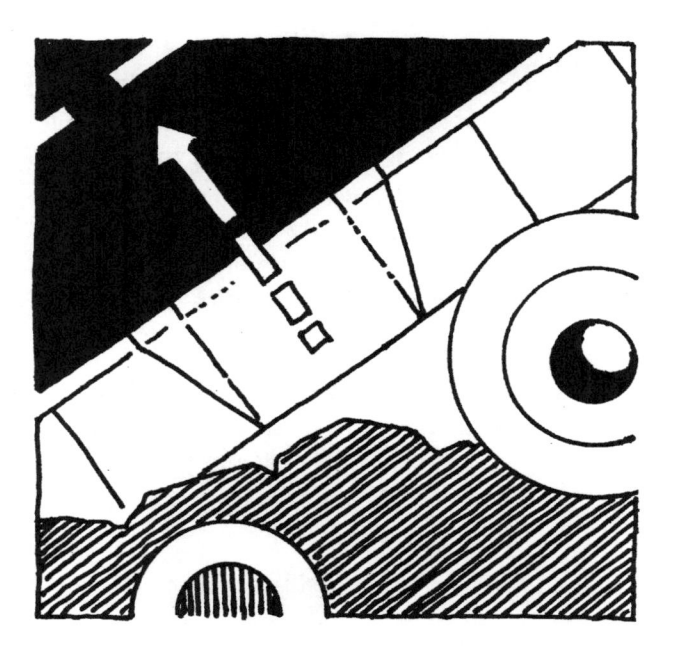

Special Circumstances

CHAPTER 5

In this Chapter

5.1	Planning Your Route	104
5.2	Crossing Streets	106
5.3	Nighttime Safety	110
5.4	Hiking	113
5.5	Traveling	116
5.6	Weather	119
5.7	Transportation	122

As you become familiar with using your wheelchair, you might want to use it in circumstances other than the controlled environments previously described. This chapter addresses some of those situations. You will likely discover other useful techniques on your own.

Read the warnings on page xi to learn about the risks involved in performing wheelchair skills. Falling is an unacceptable option for some wheelchair riders that may result in severe injury or death.

Chapter Five: Special Circumstances

Section 5.1

Planning Your Route

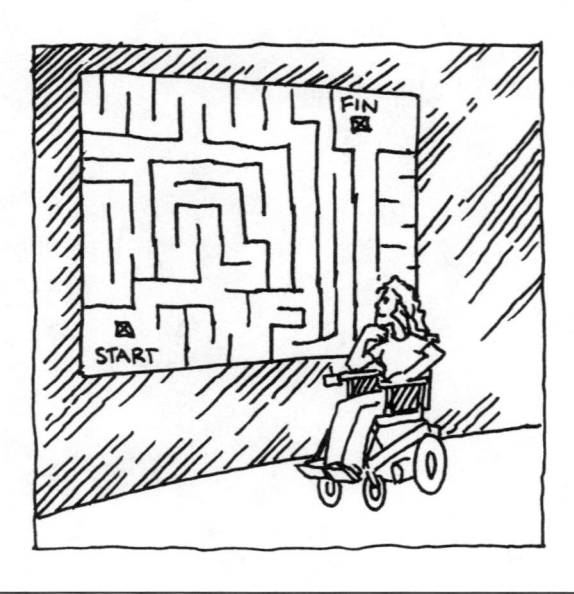

Pilots file flight plans that specify where the plane will be flying and when it is supposed to land. When planes do not arrive at their stated destinations, search parties know where to start looking. File a "flight plan" for your trips. Although you might not be used to informing others of your travel plans, it is a good idea to start now because you are using a mechanical device that can break down. Help will arrive more quickly if others are aware of your plans. This section covers the issues related to planning for the environment of travel. Section 5.7 on transportation covers more of the details of traveling.

When creating your "flight plan," try to anticipate some of the various circumstances you might have to cope with when traveling. Consider the following questions and suggestions as they correspond with the following modes of travel.

Transit Stops
- Is there a route to transit stops that is free of curbs or stairs?
- Are there ramps or elevators from the parking area or sidewalk to the transit station and loading area?
- Can you roll across the transit stop surface easily, or will you get stuck?
- How big is the loading area?
- Is there a shelter that can accommodate you?

Section 5.1: Planning Your Route

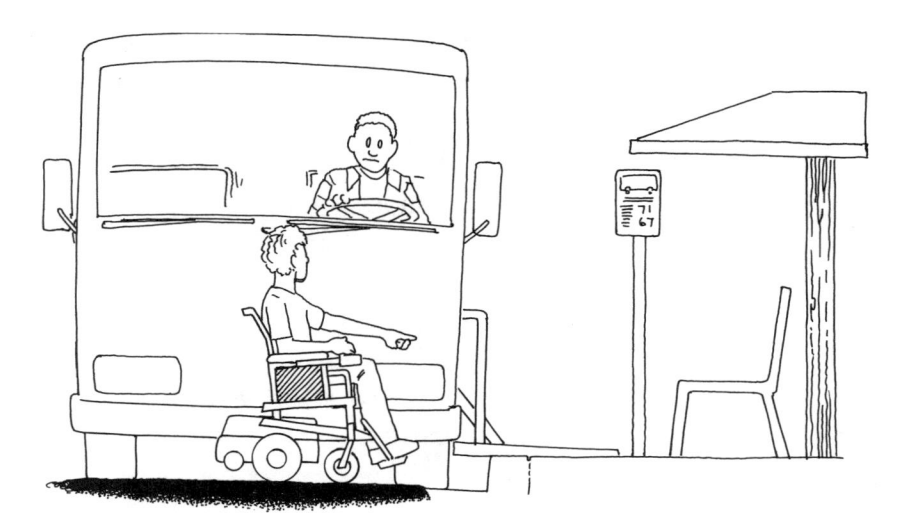

Check accessibility of loading areas for public transportation.

Airplanes

- Advise the reservation agent that you use a wheelchair.
- Request to sit in a row of seats where the armrest on the aisle lifts up out of the way to make it easier for you to transfer into the seat.
- Indicate whether or not you will be able to walk to your seat or if you will need assistance and/or an aisle chair.
- Ask the airline if the particular aircraft you are flying on has an onboard wheelchair that you could use to get to the plane's restroom.
- Pack sealed gel cell batteries or you might have to leave them behind and purchase new ones at your destination.
- Have the name and phone number of a reliable Rehabilitation Technology Supplier at your destination in case you need any repairs upon arrival.

Trains and Automobiles

- Can you board the vehicle without having to transfer out of your chair? For example, are there lifts for the bus, a drop-off or rise to board a train car, or a ramp to the airplane rather than boarding stairs?
- Are there appropriate wheelchair tiedown areas, or will you have to transfer to a seat?
- Does the transit district offer lift-equipped vehicles for people with disabilities?
- Are all vehicles on the route wheelchair accessible? Find out when and where you can catch an accessible vehicle.

Rental Vehicles

- What features in your personal vehicle would you need in a rental? Most car rental companies have left and right hand controls that can be installed in a rental car. Alternate acceleration pedals are sometimes available that can be added to almost any car if you have function in only the left leg.
- If possible, make reservations for an accessible vehicle well in advance of your trip. Most companies require at least 48 hours advance notice to install adaptive driving equipment.
- If you are using a van, ask if the vehicle has wheelchair tiedown areas, or whether you will have to transfer to a seat in the vehicle.
- Re-confirm your vehicle reservation just prior to your departure.

Chapter Five: Special Circumstances

Section 5.2

Crossing Streets

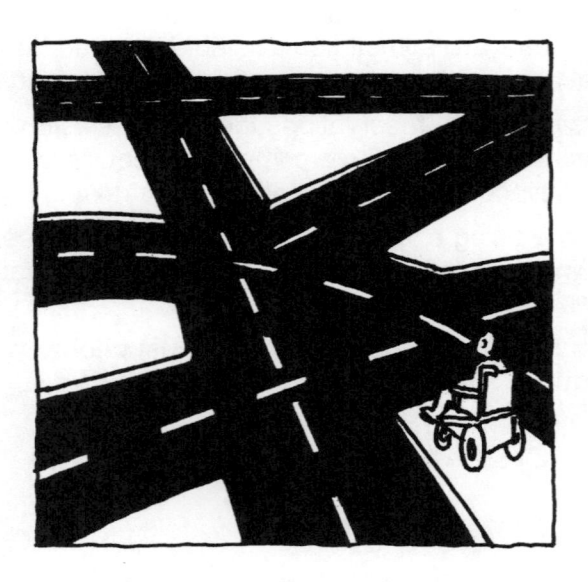

Watch for motorized vehicles, bicycles, and other pedestrians when you cross streets. Try to use a crosswalk, but remember that many motorists are unaccustomed to looking for pedestrians below eye level and that crosswalks without traffic lights are often ignored by drivers.

Before practicing the skills in this chapter, you should be able to drive a wheelchair forward and backward, cross obstacles and rough terrain, and travel up and down curb ramps and small curbs.

Always use a spotter or ask someone for help if you feel uncomfortable crossing a particular street. Ask your spotter to walk next to you as you cross the street. A spotter will be taller and, thus, more visible to motorists. A spotter can also help you maintain your balance if you have difficulty with your trunk stability.

Understand the Local Driver Mentality

In some places, motorists are more aggressive and less likely to stop for pedestrians. If you are a local resident, you will probably already be familiar with the prevailing driver mentality. If you are visiting an area for the first time, spend a few moments observing interactions between motorists and pedestrians. You may also want to ask other pedestrians about their experiences with local drivers.

Examining Street Terrain

Study the conditions of the street before you cross.
- Are there drainage grates?
- Is the road well paved or does it have potholes or bumpy surfaces?
- Are reflectors embedded in the asphalt?
- Is the surface wet or icy?
- If you need to negotiate obstacles, is there enough room to maneuver around them?

Section 5.2: Crossing Streets

- Check for vehicles, bicyclists or others turning right at red lights, as well as other pedestrians. Watch for turning vehicles even when crossing one-way streets, as some states permit drivers on a one-way street to turn left on a red light into another one-way street.
- Determine how you will move from the sidewalk to the street. Is there a curb ramp? If so, how can you best approach it? If not, can you descend the curb by yourself?
- Plan how best to ascend the sidewalk on the other side of the street. Is there a curb ramp, or will you need to climb the curb?
- Is there a center median? If so, is the median surface cut through to permit you to wait in the protected area, should you not have enough time to cross? If the median has not been cut through, is there a safe space around the median for you to wait for a signal change?
- Once in the crosswalk, establish yourself by making eye contact with motorists and cyclists, or edging forward so that motorists know you intend to cross the street.
- Wait until all vehicles have recognized your presence and have stopped to let you cross.
- As you cross the street, keep an eye on the oncoming traffic.

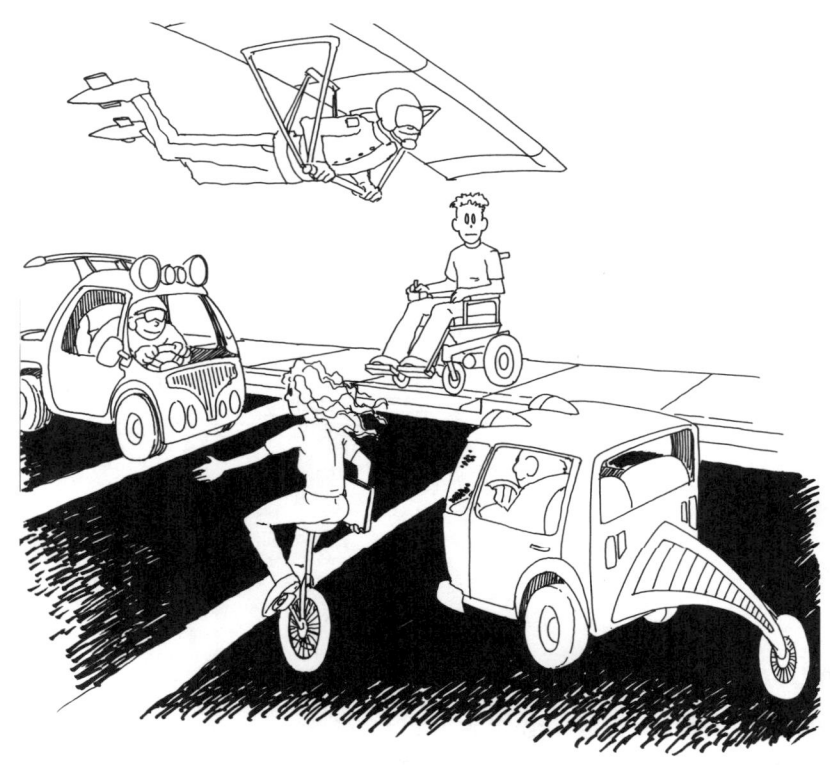

Knowing how local drivers tend to act will help you know what to expect from traffic.

Crossing at a Crosswalk

- Always try to cross at a traffic light. Be extra cautious if there is no traffic light.
- If there is a light, try timing the street crossing interval to see if you can make it to the other side before the light changes.
- Look both ways before crossing the street. Some countries, such as the United Kingdom, Australia, and Japan, drive on the left side of the road. Be especially wary when crossing streets in these countries because you might forget which way to look first.

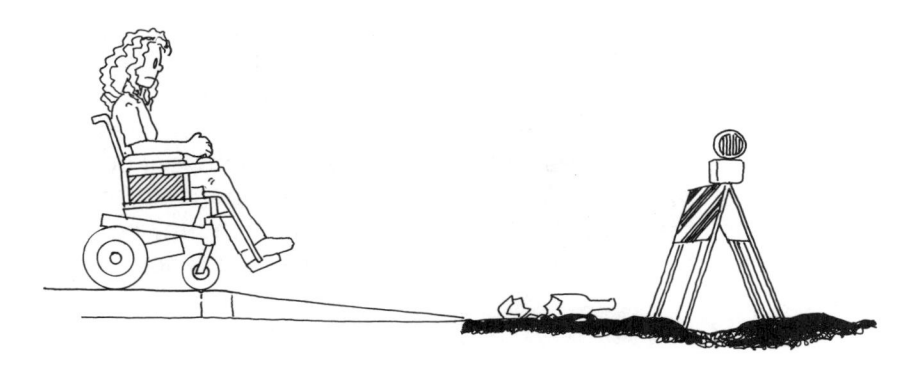

Check the condition of the crosswalk before you start across.

Chapter Five: Special Circumstances

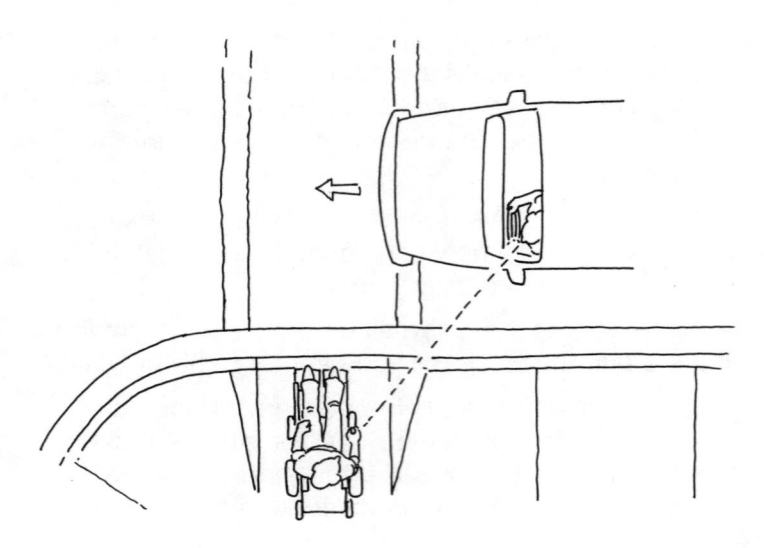

Establish eye contact so others know your intentions.

Avoid crossing between parked cars.

Crossing at Mid-block

- Avoid crossing between parked cars, because drivers cannot see you very well.
- Some smaller intersections do not have marked crosswalks. In these instances, it is safest to proceed further down the street until you reach a marked crosswalk, even if you have to backtrack down the other side of the street to get to your destination. Some small towns along two-lane state highways do not have crosswalks. This is a situation that will require extreme caution to cross the roadway. The safest solution may be to get back into your vehicle and drive it across the road.

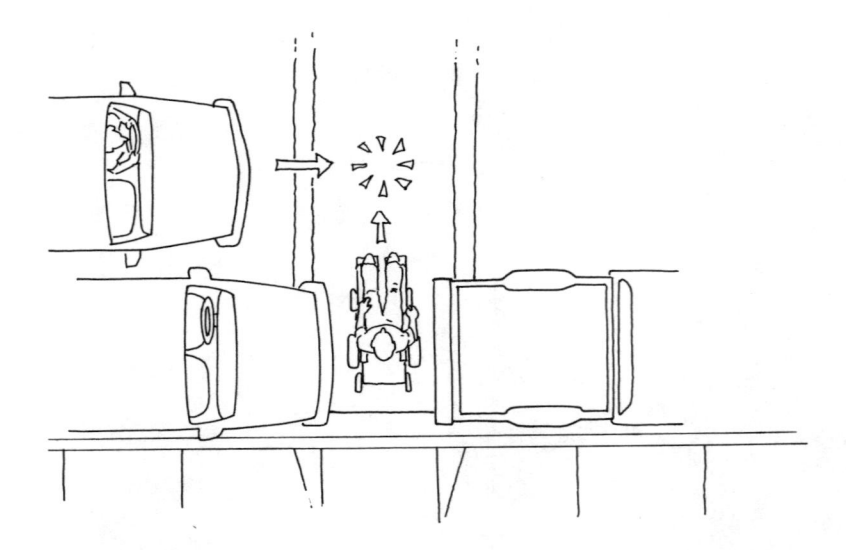

How to ask for assistance

If a road is very busy and/or it is apparent that motorists are failing to notice you, try asking for assistance.

- Look for another group crossing the street and move with them, or ask another pedestrian to walk with you as you cross. A group of people will be more visible to motorists, bicyclists, and other pedestrians. Be sure to use caution. There may be safety in numbers, but you should still be aware of traffic.
- Accessories such as flags, reflectors, bright clothing and noisemakers can improve your visibility to motorists.

How a spotter can help

- Walk next to the wheelchair rider while crossing the street.
- Keep yourself and the wheelchair rider visible to motorists.
- Prevent the upper body of the wheelchair rider from falling forward if the chair comes to an abrupt stop.

> ## Helpful Hints
>
> - Remember that in a wheelchair you are most likely shorter, thus, less visible than you would be standing up.
>
> - An accessory such as a flag can help make you more visible.
>
> - Sometimes making your intentions known can help – if you hang back on the sidewalk, motorists may not realize you want to cross. Try edging your chair down the curb ramp to the edge of the street. Do not just drive out into the street; use caution to be sure that the motorists see you and will stop to let you cross.

Driving in the street

You should have all of the rights and privileges of a pedestrian in a powered wheelchair as long as you do not drive in a reckless manner that would endanger other pedestrians. Your wheelchair was most likely set up for you to operate in a pedestrian environment. Going into the street is another matter. You would be trying to operate on the side of the roadway in a bicycle environment without the speed and maneuverability of a bicycle.

If you drive your wheelchair along the side of the road, you are taking an extreme risk. Your wheelchair does not have the speed or maneuverability to compete in this environment with other motor vehicles. A walking or running pedestrian at least has the ability to step off to the side of the road when a vehicle comes by. This may not be an option for you as a wheelchair user if there is a curb along side the road. On roads with shoulders, there may not be a large enough shoulder outside the boundary of the lane designated with striping for vehicular traffic. Vehicles often stray out of the traffic lane where they are supposed to be driving, due to distractions or the effects of alcohol or other substance abuse. Many manual and powered wheelchair users have been killed while driving on the street. Some wheelchair users have gotten tickets for driving on the street when there are sidewalks. There may be a route that you need to travel that does not have pedestrian access. Try to locate alternate routes with sidewalk access. You can also consult your pedestrian coordinator at your local city or county planning office. They may be able to correct the problem.

See further comments on this situation in the next section, Nighttime Safety.

Chapter Five: Special Circumstances

Section 5.3

Nighttime Safety

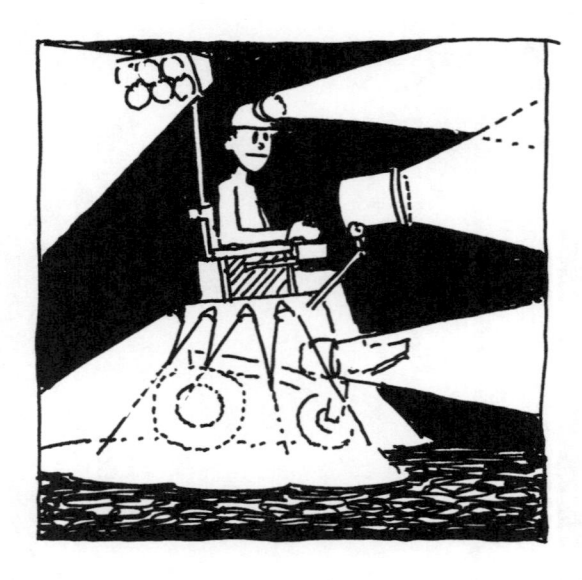

While you should always be concerned with maintaining your visibility and personal safety, you should take extra precautions when traveling at night. Darkness makes you more vulnerable to traffic accidents, as well as crime. This does not mean that you should never go out after dark. But it does mean that you should compensate for low visibility and pay careful attention to surface conditions in the dark. Always stay aware of your surroundings.

Avoid potentially hazardous situations such as very heavy traffic or unlit streets. In a wheelchair, you cannot jump out of the path of oncoming vehicles as quickly as others. Your ability to move sideways quickly to escape oncoming vehicles is most severely compromised. Remember that pedestrians walking in crosswalks are hit by vehicles every day. In fact, 30% of all traffic fatalities involve pedestrians. Powered wheelchair users are, unfortunately, included in these statistics. Be especially safety conscious when traveling near vehicles moving at high speeds.

General Pointers

Increasing your visibility to others is of prime consideration when traveling at night. When operating your wheelchair as a pedestrian in pedestrian environments such as crosswalks, you should not feel obligated to reflectorize yourself. Pedestrians have the right of way in crosswalks and it is not a requirement to reflectorize yourself. If all pedestrians were required to reflectorize themselves, then you would be required to do so as well. However, you should be extra cautious at night, especially if the crosswalk is not well lit.

You can choose to make yourself more visible by installing reflectors on the side of your wheelchair or on the wheels. This is, however, a personal choice.

- Consider your path of travel. Is it safe and well-lit? If not, can you take an alternate route?
- Make sure someone knows you are going out and where you are going. If you are traveling and will be going out alone, inform the hotel concierge or front desk of your plans and when you expect to be back.
- Call someone at your destination to let them know you are on your way and when you expect to arrive.

Driving in the street at night

If you drive your wheelchair along the side of the road at night, you are taking an extreme risk. Your wheelchair does not have the speed or maneuverability to compete in this environment with other motor vehicles. A walking or running pedestrian at least has the ability to step off to the side of the road when a vehicle comes by. This may not be an option for you as a wheelchair user if there is a curb alongside the road. On roads with shoulders, there may not be a large enough shoulder outside the boundary of the lane designated with striping for vehicular traffic. Vehicles often stray out of the traffic lane, due to distractions or the effects of alcohol or other substance abuse. Many manual and powered wheelchair users have been killed while driving on the street. If a pedestrian must travel along the side of the road, travel against the flow of traffic is generally advised.

If you must operate your wheelchair in the roadway, you should prepare your wheelchair as much as possible with respect to reflectorization and lighting. In Germany, for example, you are required by law to meet specific reflectorization and lighting requirements to drive your powered wheelchair in the street. Red taillights, a white headlight and amber running lights are standard. Reflectors must also be on the wheelchair (red on the rear and amber on the sides). Flashing light emitting diodes (LEDs) are bright and will help get the attention of motorists. You can get lighting equipment at a bicycle shop if you foresee this type of wheelchair usage. The equipment should be permanently installed with a switch so you can turn the lighting on and off independently.

Wearing shoes or clothing with reflectorization, like runners often do, will help when operating in a street environment at night. However, this is not a substitute for the use of a full lighting package.

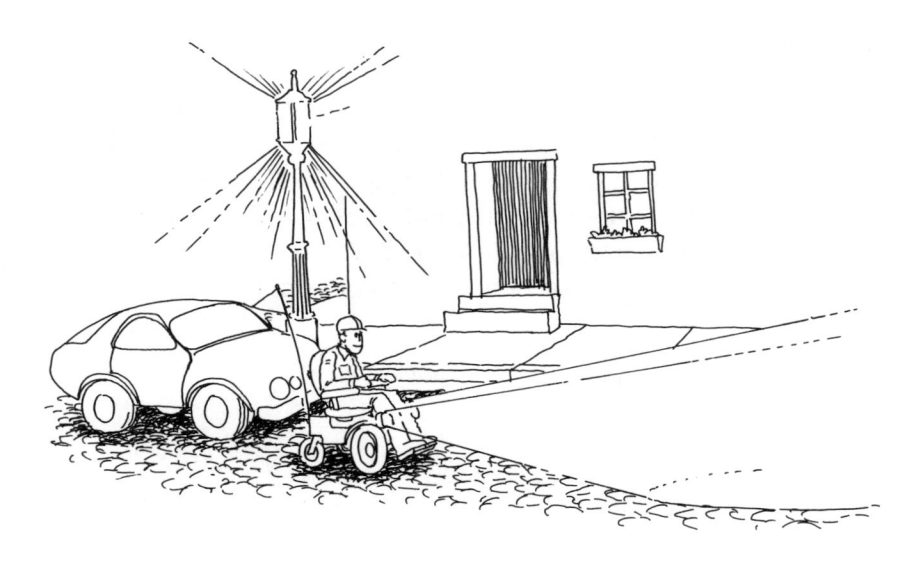

Reflectors and lights may increase your visibility at night if you must operate in the street with other motor vehicles.

Emergency Equipment

Always be prepared for emergencies. You do not need to bring a police dog, flares and your entire set of socket wrenches, however. Here is a list of a few things that are indispensable in most emergencies:

- a flashlight
- a patch kit and tire pump
- a cellular phone
- a whistle or other noisemaker to attract attention

Protect Yourself

Take a self-defense course. People might pick on you even though, and perhaps because, you use a wheelchair. Make sure the class includes verbal, as well as physical self-defense. Some self-defense courses are designed specifically for women, while others are geared toward people with disabilities. Some classes specifically address the use of mace and/or pepper sprays.

Moving Around

Sidewalks

- Stay on well-lit sidewalks so you can see obstacles.

Curbs

- Try to climb curbs where there is enough light so you can see obstacles more easily.

Parking

Drive the route from where you are going to where you will park during the daylight, so you can determine the best route to drive your wheelchair.

- Try to park in well-lit areas.
- Make sure there is enough room to enter and exit your vehicle.
- If you parallel park your vehicle on a street, be sure that your lift will unload onto the sidewalk and not into the street.

Section 5.4

Hiking

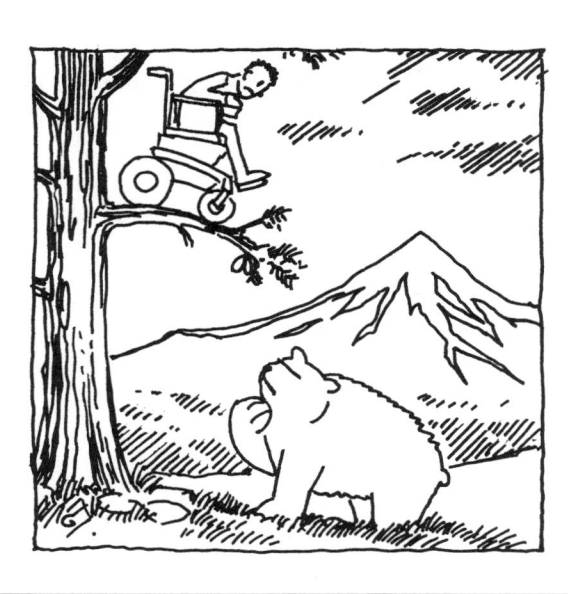

Hiking Hazards

Outdoor environments can present major challenges to wheelchair navigation. Unpaved natural surfaces, steep grades, and wild vegetation make trails both scenic and challenging to access.

When hiking, watch for:

- Sections of the trail that are very steep (see Section 3.5 for more information about how to navigate steep slopes).
- Sections of the trail with a steep side slope (see Section 3.6 for more information about cross slopes).
- Soft surfaces (see Section 3.4 for more information about rough terrain).
- Narrow spots on the trail (see Section 3.3 for more information about navigating in tight environments).
- Obstacles such as rocks, ruts, and roots (see Section 3.2 for more information about navigating over and around obstacles).

Prepare for Your Trip

Try to find out as much information as possible about a trail before you hike it. The information will help you plan a hike that meets your needs, whether you are looking for leisure enjoyment, a physical challenge, or anything else. Information about the following trail characteristics may be helpful:

- Length of the trail – Do you have enough battery power?
- Average and maximum grade
- Average and maximum cross slope
- Average and minimum width
- Trail surface type and condition
- Obstacles that may exist on the trail

Chapter Five: Special Circumstances

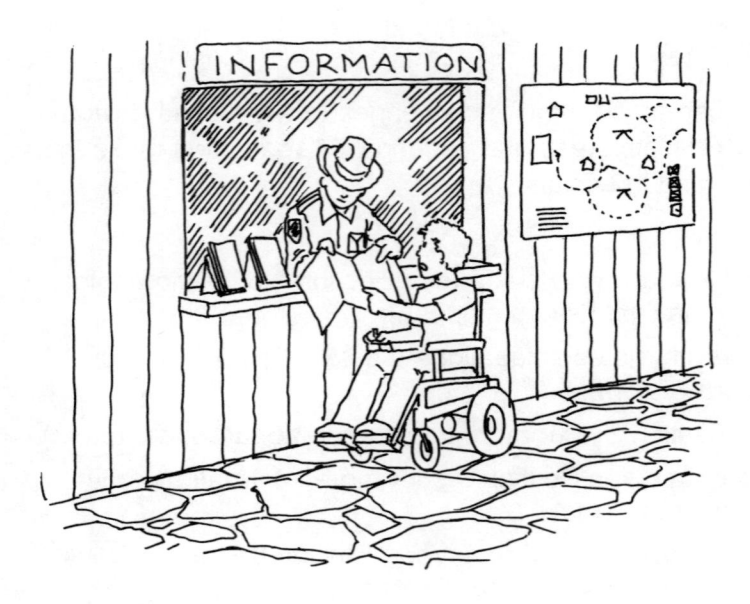

Learn about the trail before you start hiking it.

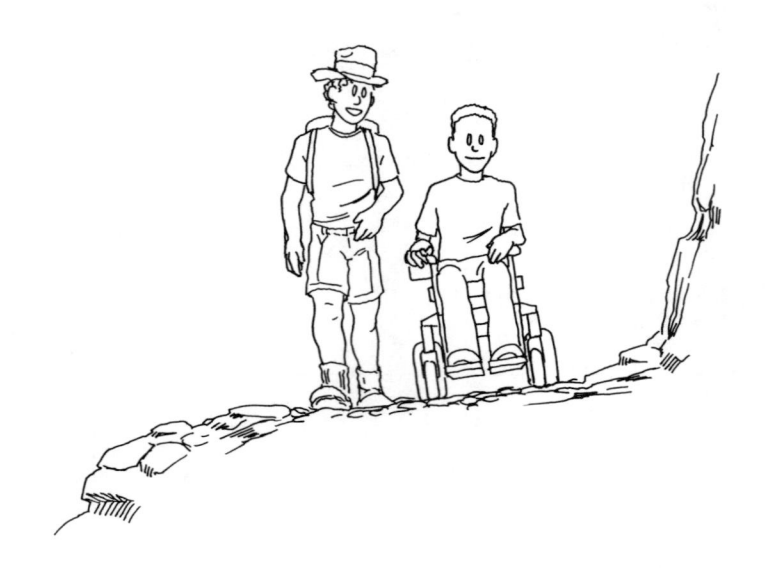

Have your spotter walk along the downhill side of the trail where they will be able to assist more easily.

Take Precautions

- Be prepared for emergencies. Carry a cellular phone or a hand held radio for emergency communication.
- Do not hike by yourself in your wheelchair. Unlike most other people, you cannot walk out if your wheels break down.

Asking for Assistance

You may need assistance from others if you encounter difficult spots along your hike.

Narrow sections with drop-offs

- Ask your spotter to walk on the downhill side of the trail.
- You may want your spotter to hold on to your chair as you travel through narrow sections of the trail.

Rocks, ruts, roots and other obstacles

- Ask your spotter to support your chair from the side or rear while you are attempting to cross the obstacle.
- The spotter can help you cross an obstacle by pushing down and forward on the push handles to unweight the casters.

Section 5.4: Hiking

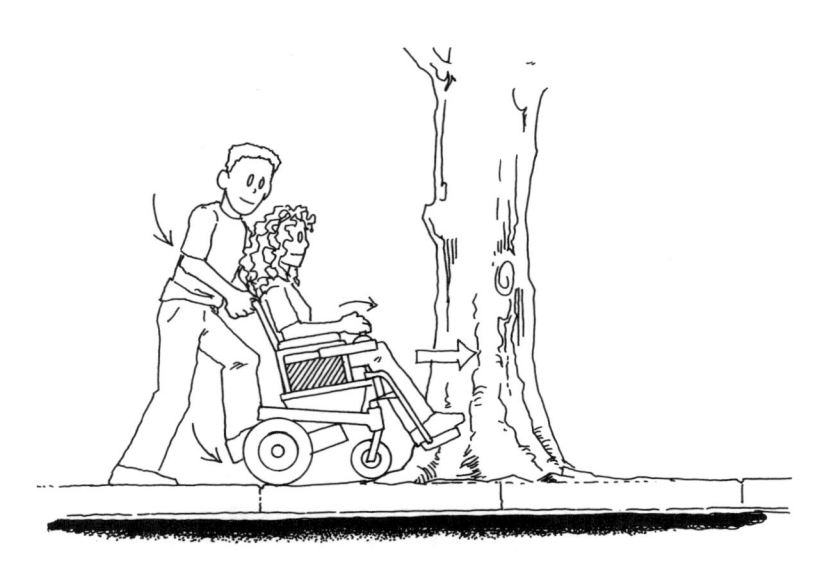

By pushing down and forward on the push handles, a spotter can help unweight the casters.

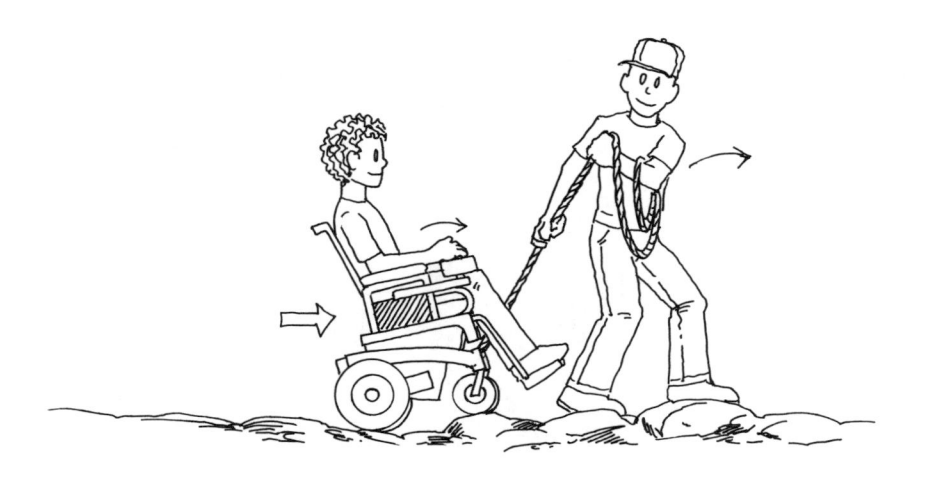

Tying a rope to the front of the wheelchair can enable someone to assist you. The rope can be used to pull the front casters up over obstructions, and to pull forward to assist with going up a steep trail.

Going up and down hills

- If getting assistance with a tow rope is something you are willing to do, carry one or two pieces of strong rope or webbing at least 15 feet long.
- The rope or webbing can be tied to a solid portion of the wheelchair's front frame to enable an assistant to pull or stabilize you when navigating a difficult section of the trail.
- Experiment with different rope attachment points to find a spot where a tow will unweight your front casters but will not tip you back. If the attachment point is too low, the towing force will lift the front of the chair too high and flip you over backward.
- Lean forward as you are being towed to avoid tipping backward out of your chair.
- Rope or webbing can also be attached to a low part of the frame on the rear of the wheelchair, to help slow your descent on steep sections of the trail.

CAUTION

Attaching rope or webbing up high on the rear of the wheelchair could tip the chair backward. Be sure to attach rope or webbing to a low part of the frame.

Section 5.5

Traveling

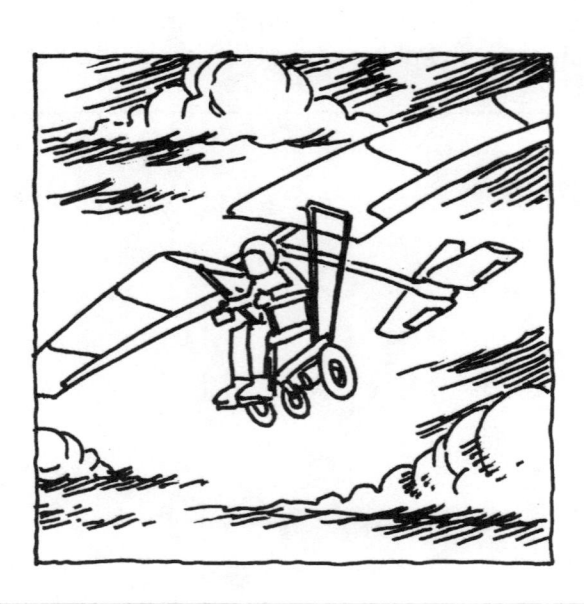

Have you ever looked forward to a fabulous meal at a great restaurant, dressed in your best, and fought your way onto the bus, or endured a heart-stopping taxi van ride, only to find the place located up a flight of stairs? Sometimes it's not a lack of access but a lack of information that will make your journey difficult. Taking a few minutes to call ahead can solve lots of problems and save lots of time in the long run. Be specific when asking questions; someone else's idea of "accessible" may be very different from yours. Don't be surprised if you are told a restaurant is accessible even if it occupies the upper floor of a building without an elevator. If a destination you have been told is accessible turns out to be inaccessible, request an interview with the facility manager. Tell the manager that "accessible" means an environment in compliance with the Americans with Disabilities Act (ADA) Accessibility Guidelines, and that your inability to use the facility probably indicates the establishment needs to improve its access measures. Appendix A contains more information about the ADA.

Note: All commercial entities must make a reasonable accommodation to provide access to persons with disabilities. A reasonable accommodation is determined according to the financial resources of the entity which owns the establishment.

Travel Planning Tips

Part of the appeal of going to new places is the fun of exploring the unknown. Though you may think advance reconnaissance is cheating and dull, it is usually worthwhile to obtain basic access information about the site to avoid disappointment and frustration. You don't want to arrive at a wedding, dressed in nice clothing, only to find you must cross a muddy path to get to the reception. Nor would it be amusing to arrive at a hotel and discover the "accessible guest room" has a shower stall sized to accommodate slender people but not you and your shower chair. Make a practice of calling ahead of time and talking to friends or acquaintances who have been there before.

Consider asking the following questions:

- What kinds of obstacles will you face in route to your destination? Are there elevators or stairs? Do the curbs have ramps? Will someone be there to help you over the lawn that's been transformed into a snow field?
- Is the route all indoors, or is a portion of it outside?
- Are there ramps or elevators leading to different levels of the destination? Are the elevators or stairway lifts working? Are there signs to indicate the location of elevators and ramps?

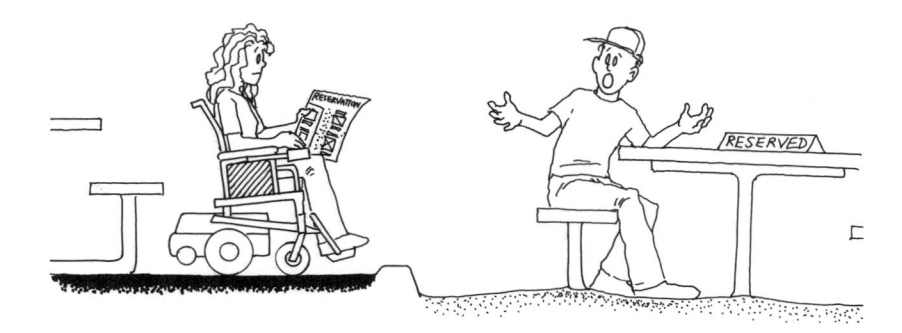

Calling ahead, on your way to an event, could save you frustration.

Hotel Rooms

- Is there a wheelchair-accessible room? What floor is it on? Is there an elevator?
- How wide is the door leading to the room? What kind of knobs, handles, or latches does it have?
- How big is the bathroom? How wide is the door? Does it swing in or out? Is there a bathtub or a roll-in shower? Where is the door in relation to the toilet and bathtub? Are there grab bars? Are the towels placed within reach?
- Can you move furniture out of the way to make it more accessible? If you do move furniture, let the housekeeping staff know you don't want it put back in place each morning. You may also be able to arrange for the actual removal of unneeded furniture from the room.
- Can you move the bed to position the wheelchair next to it for transfers? Some hotel beds are on an immovable pedestal that has no provision to roll a lift mechanism underneath the bed.
- Can you reach the temperature controls and drapery cords?
- Is the telephone within easy reach from the bed? Is the TV remote control moveable or is it bolted down? If it is fixed to the bedside table, it may be out of reach.
- If your hotel room poses access problems, try brainstorming solutions with the management. For example, ask them to wrap and tape towels around exposed hot water pipes under sinks. Another common request is to remove the bathroom door if the opening is too narrow for your wheelchair, or if the door blocks access to other elements of the bathroom.

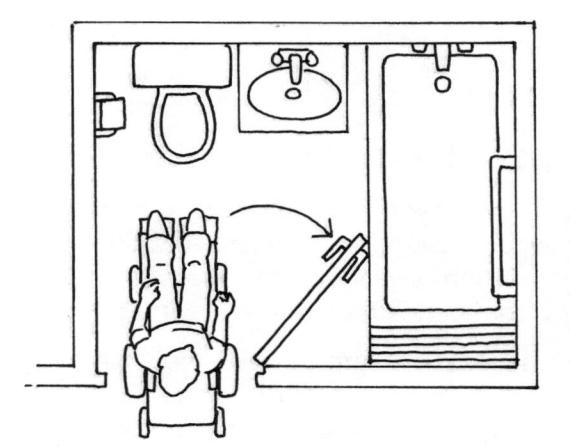

This bathtub would be usable if the bathroom door could swing out. Asking the management to remove the door might be a temporary solution.

Restrooms

- Is the restroom on the same floor as your destination (e.g. meeting room, reception, etc.)?
- How wide is the restroom doorway? Does the door open in or out? Can it be opened in a single motion (e.g. swinging door, pull handle)?

Chapter Five: Special Circumstances

- How big is the restroom? Is there room to maneuver inside? How big is the stall?
- Are there grab bars?

New Environments

Your capabilities will vary depending on your environment. For example, wheeling around a rural mid-western town is very different from trying to navigate and get around independently in New York City. Many factors affect wheelchair mobility, including:

- Upkeep of sidewalks and streets
- Availability of curb ramps
- Weather conditions (e.g. snow, ice, humidity, rain)
- Traffic laws (e.g. Do pedestrians have the right of way? Can motorists make a right turn on a red light?)
- Crowds

> ### Helpful Hints
>
> If you have room when you travel, you could bring a sturdy webbed beach chair or folding chair with you. It can be used as a shower chair. Alternatively, you can use a chair from the dining room, conference room, or bedroom.
>
> Know your rights to access! Be familiar with the ADA (Americans with Disabilities Act) Accessibility Guidelines and get a feel for what might be a reasonable accommodation in any given situation.

Other Hazards

Be aware of heat sources that may be near your feet. If you feel any warmth coming up from anywhere around you, feel along your pants for excessive heat or ask someone to feel if parts of your body that you cannot reach could be in danger of getting burned.

Section 5.6

Weather

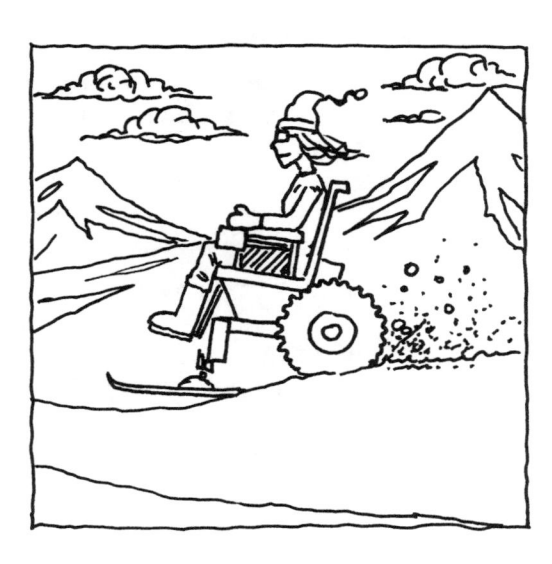

Weather and its residues impact your ability to use your wheelchair. For example, on a windy day, you might feel your wheelchair being pushed by the wind and have to compensate to keep going straight. Depending on where you live, it might be useful to learn to negotiate snow banks and icy surfaces, as well as rain puddles and mud. Have a spotter walk beside your wheelchair the first few times you encounter a new weather condition. Your spotter should be ready to prevent your upper body from falling forward if you lose your balance and to help get your wheelchair out if you get stuck.

Consider the following before traveling in bad weather:

- Be prepared before you go outside. Are you wearing the proper clothing? Are your tires in good condition? Do you have a flashlight?
- Think about the route you plan to take. Does your path require you to cross terrain that will be difficult in current weather conditions? Is there an alternative route that would be safer and/or easier?

Precipitation

- Keep extra rain and snow gear in places you spend a lot of time, such as your home, car or office. This way you will be prepared for any weather conditions.
- Consider using a poncho-style slicker with a hood. This versatile piece of outerwear will help keep you dry and can be positioned to cover items you need to carry on your lap. Tuck the slicker's edges under your legs to avoid catching the fabric in your wheels.
- Clothing guards can help protect your clothes from getting splattered with mud and water.
- A hat with a wide brim can prevent the rain and snow from dripping down your neck.
- Gloves with a grip are good for keeping your hands warm and dry, and to keep your hand from sliding off your joystick.

Rain

- Look at the surface ahead of you as you move around in rainy weather.
- Be cautious of obstacles, such as grates, that might be hiding under puddles, particularly at curb ramps.

- Puddles can be deeper than they look.
- Observe pedestrians crossing the same area before initiating your own crossing.
- Remember that some wet surfaces are slippery. Moving slowly will help you stay in control. Even if you are on a familiar surface, it will be more slippery than when it is dry.

Ice, snow and slush

After a snowstorm, a familiar area may look entirely different. There may be uneven surfaces due to packed snow and melting ice. Passages may be narrower because of the accumulation of snow and snow banks, and hazards, such as grates and curbs, can be concealed under a uniform blanket of white. When approaching an intersection, both your visibility and the visibility of motorists will be greatly reduced, and motorists may not see you drive across the street. Remember to allow yourself extra time to travel through hazardous conditions.

The type of tires you use affects how you move on ice. Pneumatic and treaded tires grip surfaces better than solid or ribbed tires.

- Look at the surface ahead of you as you move around in snow, ice or slushy conditions. Check for icy patches and for obstacles, such as grates, that might be hidden under snow or slush, particularly at curb ramps. Slush is often deeper than it looks. Observe pedestrians crossing the same area.
- Proceed slowly on icy surfaces.
- Slush and snow will act much like the rough terrain of sand and gravel. Watch your caster position when changing directions to avoid getting stuck. Keep both casters pointed in the same direction for maximum stability.

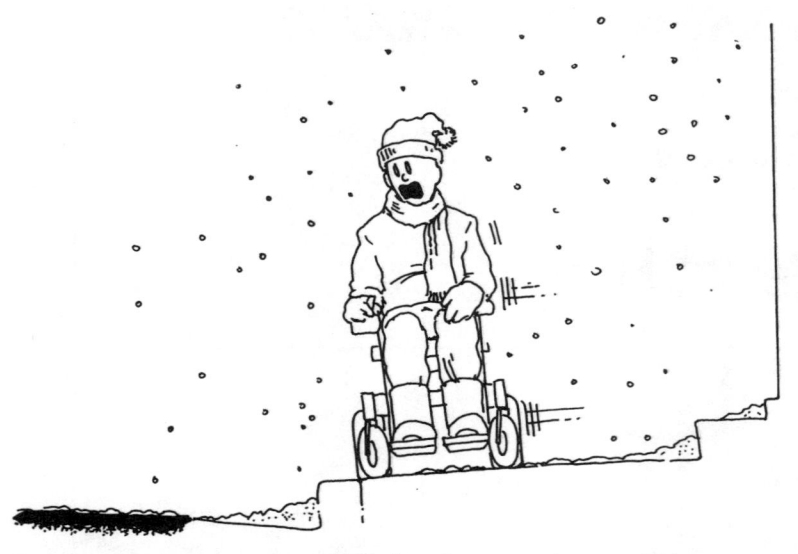

Keeping your momentum may help when crossing small icy patches; but whenever you can, avoid driving on ice.

Traveling in snow with an assistant

- Should your casters sink into snow, you could ask an assistant to push down and forward on the push handles to unweight your casters as you drive forward.
- Alternatively, have an assistant tie a rope to the front of the wheelchair to help guide you. If attached near the front wheels/casters, pulling on the rope will unweight the front casters, making it easier to drive through the snow.

CAUTION

Attaching rope or webbing up high on the rear of the wheelchair could tip the chair backward. Be sure to attach rope or webbing to a low part of the frame.

Sun

If you live in a place that gets hot or humid, consider the following:

- Keep loose and light clothing handy.
- Keep a hat in your clothing stash to shade your eyes from the sun, and a sweatband or bandanna to keep the sweat out of your eyes.
- Sunglasses can protect your eyes from the sun and limit glare.
- Carry a water bottle with you at all times, especially in the summer.
- If your sensation is impaired in the lower extremities, be careful not to burn yourself. Touch the lower frame of your wheelchair with your arm or hand to see if it is hot. If your wheelchair has been stored in the sun, van or other hot area, the metal can get very hot.

Wind

- Keep long hair tied back when venturing into very windy weather. This will help keep your hair out of your eyes.
- Eyeglasses and sunglasses can keep dirt from blowing in your eyes.
- Look at the surface ahead of you as you navigate your chair in windy weather. Be cautious of obstacles that might have blown onto the surface.
- In strong wind, you may need to compensate with the control input device to maintain a straight path.

How a spotter can help

- Walk on the non-joystick side of the wheelchair. Be ready to catch the upper body of the wheelchair rider if the casters get stuck and balance is lost.

Section 5.7
Transportation

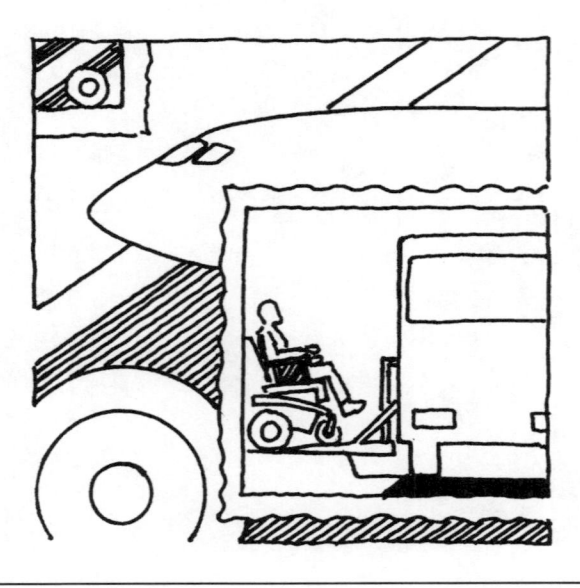

General Considerations and Safety Issues

For most users, to function effectively in today's society, both for work and for pleasure, your powered wheelchair will not be the only method of transportation you need. However, using other methods of transportation with your powered wheelchair, such as motor vehicles, trains, and airplanes, can be more than tricky at times. You need to plan your strategy ahead of time to ensure that your travel is safe and without problems. In most cases, and especially in private motor vehicle transportation, the safest way to travel is by transferring to the vehicle's original seat, although there are some exceptions. When you transfer to the seat of a private motor vehicle, you are able to use the occupant restraint system (seat belts and airbags) and seating that has been crash-tested and complies with federal motor vehicle safety standards.

If you need additional support to stay upright, add straps, belts or other postural supports. Some seatbacks recline, which is a feature that might improve your trunk balance in the forward direction. However, you should be aware that reclining more than 35 degrees can reduce the effectiveness of the safety belts in a frontal crash, so do not recline more than necessary.

The first thing you will need to do before traveling is to make the decision whether or not you can, or will, transfer from your wheelchair into another seat. For some powered wheelchair users, the option to independently transfer does not exist. When traveling on aircraft, transferring out of your wheelchair is mandatory. Airports usually have trained personnel to assist you in making the transfer from your powered wheelchair to an aisle wheelchair that can move down the aisle of the airplane. Most public bus and van transportation systems do not provide the assistance needed to transfer into the vehicle seats. In private vans and other personal vehicles, the assistance required to transfer may not be available either.

For most powered wheelchair users who cannot transfer independently, you will need to ride in private or public transportation vehicles while sitting in your wheelchair. It is important to understand what the safety issues are so you can make intelligent decisions about whether you want to try to transfer or remain seated in your wheelchair.

This section of the book briefly discusses specific issues and safety considerations that will come up with regard to transferring or remaining in your powered wheelchair when using different modes of transportation, including:

- Automobiles and taxis
- Personal and public vans
- Buses and trains
- Air travel

Transferring In and Out of Your Wheelchair

During motor vehicle transportation, and especially in private vehicles, it is almost always safer to be sitting in the seat that was designed for that vehicle, using the lap and shoulder belts that comply with federal safety standards. However, in some cases, you may not be able to achieve the necessary postural support while seated in a vehicle seat, and may, therefore, find it more appropriate to remain seated in your wheelchair. This part of the section discusses various transportation issues that you will need to consider when transferring in and out of your wheelchair and using the vehicle seat. For some powered wheelchair users, transferring in and out of your wheelchair may present hazards and physical risks for you or the people assisting you, which makes transferring not feasible or even possible. This situation is discussed in the next part of this section.

If you plan to transfer and the transportation you need to use does not have a lift, your only choice may be to be lifted or carried into the vehicle. This usually means that your wheelchair will need to be disassembled so that it can be lifted or carried onto the vehicle separately. In this situation, you might as well be placed into seating that was designed for that vehicle and use the provided lap and shoulder restraints. Be sure to ask for your wheelchair to be properly secured so that it does not become a flying projectile in the event of an accident.

Using automobiles and taxis

Transporting your powered wheelchair in a car or taxi can be difficult or impossible. Unless your wheelchair can be taken apart or folded, it will not fit in most sedan-type vehicles. Even if your wheelchair does come apart, it may be too difficult to lift or pack into a car or taxi. Some powered wheelchairs are designed to fit more easily into a car. The batteries can be removed and the frame folded to fit into the back of a wagon or a spacious trunk. A powered wheelchair with batteries removed, but with the motor still attached, can weigh 80 pounds or more. The car will most likely need to have a lift, or be a hatchback, mini-van, SUV, or wagon with ramps to get the power base in and out of the vehicle.

Another complication with transferring for automobile travel is making the vehicle seat accommodate your needs. Putting a 1-inch gel cushion over the car seat will give you good skin protection without raising you up too high above the car seat surface. Gel cushions are usually not used much on wheelchairs because of their weight. However, if you leave the gel cushion in the car, the weight is not really an issue. If you are going to be riding for long distances, or are prone to pressure ulcers, you could also use your wheelchair cushion in the car seat. However, this may also place you too high on the seat. Some people may need to use a back support or add custom seating to the car. Be sure to always wear the car's three-point safety belt (lap and shoulder belts), as they will provide protection in an accident and will give you some extra trunk support.

Riding in a taxi will be a problem unless you can transfer to the front or rear seat of a four-door sedan. Someone else might have to take your wheelchair apart into smaller, liftable pieces to stow in the car and/or trunk. Most cities have lift-equipped taxi services that you can use. Most taxi companies require some amount of advance notice to reserve such taxis. The United Kingdom uses large taxis, some of which have ramps that enable wheelchairs to drive right into the back seat area.

Transferring to the driver seat

If you want to drive and can transfer to the driver's seat, you can have your vehicle modified so that it can be operated using special hand controls. Contact a vehicle modification professional in the community or your rehab facility to get more information about adaptive driving controls. But remember that, unless you can manage getting your wheelchair into and out of the vehicle independently, you will not be able to go places without assistance.

If you use a scooter or have partial mobility, lift platforms are available that attach to the back of a vehicle. These allow you to drive your wheelchair onto the lift, get out of your wheelchair, raise the lift, and get into the drivers seat.

Transferring and driving from a van or minivan is easier than using a sedan or pickup truck. Sometimes it is possible to get your wheelchair into a van by tipping the wheelchair into a "wheelie" position, putting the front wheels up into the van, and then lifting the back of the wheelchair in. This can sometimes be done with only one assistant. At other times, the wheelchair must be lifted or hoisted into the van by several strong people. You also might have the van equipped with a lift or an electric ramp. After getting into the van, you can transfer into the driver's seat.

Riding in Vehicles While in Your Wheelchair

Traveling in personal vehicles and vans

As previously noted, it is not always possible or feasible to transfer out of your wheelchair when traveling in a motor vehicle. In these situations, the vehicle will need to be equipped with a powered lift or ramp to assist you in getting into the vehicle in your powered wheelchair. Privately owned vans are frequently modified for use by people who use powered wheelchairs. Common modifications include adding a lift or ramp and lowering the floor or raising the roof so you have more headroom. Adding a wheelchair securement system and specialized driving controls will enable you to drive from your wheelchair. However, there are important safety concerns that need to be addressed when you remain seated in your wheelchair.

In particular, the vehicle needs to provide a way to effectively secure your wheelchair, and there needs to be a lap and shoulder belt restraint system that you can use while you are seated in your wheelchair. If your wheelchair is not properly secured to the vehicle, it could become a flying projectile, with you in it, during an accident. Also, the additional mass of the wheelchair will add to the forces on your body by the restraint system. Public transportation systems can require you to have your powered wheelchair or scooter properly secured, since failure to do so could be hazardous to yourself and others. A forward facing four-point tiedown system is the standard of the industry because it can accommodate a wide range of wheelchairs. Crash testing has shown that sitting facing sideways in a vehicle, even with a four-point tiedown system, is bad news if the vehicle makes a sudden stop or has a frontal collision! You should, therefore, always sit with your wheelchair facing forward.

If you plan to drive while seated in your wheelchair, an automatic or docking-type securement system that allows you to independently lock your wheelchair in the driving position is necessary. For these systems, special hardware must be permanently attached to your powered wheelchair that mates with hardware in the van to lock your wheelchair in. Electromagnetic switches are used to disengage the wheelchair so you can drive back out, and a manual override must be provided in case of an emergency power failure. You should attempt to verify that your wheelchair has been crash tested with the lock-down securement system that you intend to use. This information is typically available from the lock-down manufacturer.

Section 5.7: Transportation

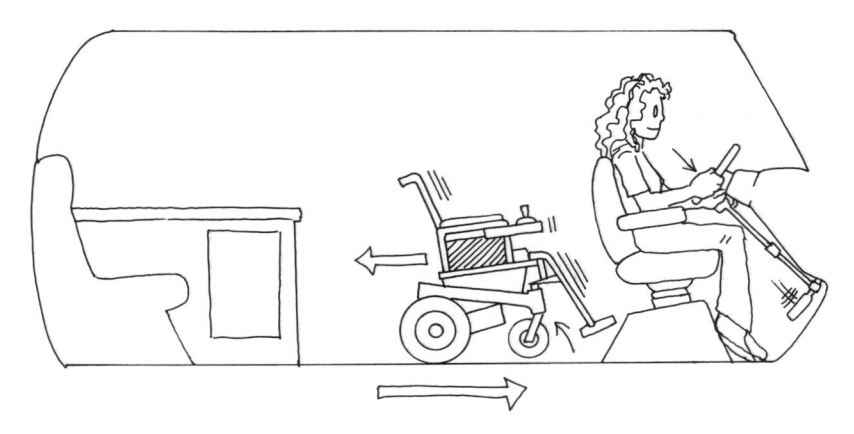

Make sure your wheelchair is secured so it does not move around as you drive.

In addition to securing your wheelchair, you should use a belt-type restraint system to keep you in your chair and from contacting the vehicle interior or other occupants. The lap belt or chest strap on your wheelchair that you use for postural support is not adequate for restraint in the event of a vehicle crash. Crash testing studies show that these postural support belts just rip right out of the chair at their attachment points, or the latching mechanisms release. When this happens, the wheelchair user goes flying forward to impact some other part of the vehicle, or possibly is ejected from the vehicle, which are the most common causes of serious and fatal injuries in car crashes.

Crash tested belt restraints should, therefore, be included with every wheelchair securing system. It is up to you to insist on them being used for your safety in the event of a crash. Be aware that a restraint around you that is attached to the floor of the vehicle without a separate wheelchair securing system will allow the wheelchair to crush you against the restraint system when it moves forward during a crash. It is important for your wheelchair to be secured AND for you to be restrained!

In order for the lap belt restraints to provide effective protection for the wheelchair user, the wheelchair must be strong enough to be secured by the tiedown system and it must provide effective seat and back support during a crash. Unfortunately, most wheelchairs have not been designed for occupancy in a motor vehicle and, therefore, may not have sufficient strength to deal with the forces of a serious crash.

Many wheelchair manufacturers are now offering transportable wheelchairs that have been crash tested while secured with four-point tiedown systems and drive-in lockdown systems. Some of these transportable wheelchairs are available with crash tested seat belts that are part of the wheelchair and with four securement attachment points that are compatible with four-point tiedown securement systems. This eliminates the requirement to have a separate restraint system to keep you in the wheelchair while being transported. A transportable wheelchair that has been crash tested will be labeled as such. The attachment points for the tiedown system will also be labeled. The next time you need to order a new wheelchair, you should ask the manufacturer if the model that you want is offered with the tested *transit option*.

If you customarily ride in a motor vehicle while seated in your wheelchair, you should also consider adding a head support to your wheelchair to reduce the possibility of head and neck injuries from aggressive starts and stops, and rear impacts. Today, all seats in motor vehicles are required to have head supports to protect riders against whiplash injury, and you might think about using one too!

There are national and international standards and procedures for testing wheelchairs designed specifically for transport in a motor vehicle. There are also test procedures to test the wheelchair securing and occupant restraint systems. Make sure you ask the manufacturers or transit company if the equipment they are selling or using complies with these standards.

Note: For more information about available specialized auto equipment, contact local rehabilitation professionals or ask for referrals from your rehabilitation facility.

Traveling in buses and trains

Accessible public transportation should be available in almost all areas of the United States. This usually means that public buses and trains are equipped with lifts and most should have wheelchair securement and occupant restraint systems. Designated buses are available on an "as needed" basis in some communities where most buses are not accessible. Contact the transportation company for more information.

Call ahead to prepare for your trip. Check to make sure the route to the bus or train station or stop is accessible. Determine the best location to purchase your tickets and find out the locations of accessible loading and unloading areas, which are often located in specific cars of a train. When using a metro train on a regular basis, you should ride the car that stops closest to your accessible route.

Most often, the seats on public transportation do not have occupant restraint belts. If there is a place for you to position and secure your wheelchair facing forward that offers occupant restraints, it is best to use this provided place. Also, if you are not comfortable with the method of wheelchair securement or occupant restraint, get off the vehicle and seek an alternate form of travel. Do not put yourself at risk unless you are willing to accept the consequences.

When traveling by train, making a reservation is a good idea. Indicate that access and use of a wheelchair accessible car is desired. Access onto trains usually requires some assistance. When the boarding platform is elevated to the same height as the car entrance, an attendant will usually place a bridging plate across the gap to allow you to roll into the car. When the boarding platform is not level with the car, a portable ramp is usually moved into place for you to enter the car. Most trains have a car with a bathroom designed for wheelchair access and a space for you to ride the train in your own wheelchair. The conductors on the train and at the stations can usually assist with your luggage and any additional assistance you might need.

Some wheelchair users argue that they do not need to use personal occupant restraint belts as seatbelts since no one else on the bus or train is using them. However, on buses, the seats in front of each seat often provide some passive restraint. If there is a passive restraint or compartment in front of the area where your wheelchair is positioned, and you are willing to accept an increased probability of injury by be being thrown into it during an accident, then you might opt to not use a seat belt. However, you still need to have your powered wheelchair secured or it will be a hazard to other occupants of the vehicle. Remember that, even though other occupants may not be using belt restraints, the seat that they are sitting on is attached securely to the vehicle and will not move about in an accident. It is also important to note that the most effective protection for you in a crash or during emergency driving maneuvers is provided through wearing occupant restraints. Experts recommend that you wear occupant restraints at all times when traveling in a motor vehicle.

Air Travel

Reservations

When making a plane reservation, let the reservation agent know that you use a wheelchair. When making a seat selection, you will not be allowed to sit in an emergency exit row. You should request to sit in a row of seats where the armrest on the aisle comes up to make it easier for you to transfer into the seat. Also indicate whether or not you will be able to walk to your seat, or if you will need assistance using the airline's aisle wheelchair to get you to your seat.

Some people prefer to sit in the aisle seat because it is the easiest to transfer into. Others prefer sliding over to the window seat so other passengers do not have to climb over them to get out. Most planes do not have accessible bathrooms, although small aisle wheelchairs are often available on the aircraft. With an onboard wheelchair, you may be able to reach the bathroom and maneuver the front of the wheelchair far enough into the doorway to use the toilet. You will need to ask the flight attendants to draw the curtains closed or clear the area to give you some privacy. On 747's there are two bathrooms across from each other and the doors open to create one large bathroom.

Preparing your wheelchair

Most airlines have experience with wheelchair users, but some may only have limited experience with people who use powered wheelchairs. Your wheelchair will probably be transported in the cargo hold. Some carriers will take your wheelchair apart to transport it, but gate checking a powered wheelchair is not a good idea. To ensure that your wheelchair is dismantled and packed properly, you should consider preparing it for transport yourself. It is wise to detach anything on your chair that is removable, such as leg supports, arm supports, and the joystick control. Packing these items in a bag on board the aircraft will ensure that you do not lose them. It also prevents them from getting damaged. Some of your seating components, such as your seat cushion, may also be useful to you on board the aircraft. You should do all of this at the ticket counter to give yourself more time at the aircraft to board. This also allows more time for your wheelchair to get on board the aircraft.

You should be aware that the airlines will generally only transport gel-cell batteries. No liquid acid-filled batteries will be accepted on the aircraft, although some carriers might remove the batteries and transport them separately in special containers. Make sure your carrier knows what type of batteries you have.

Boarding

Usually the airport personnel will transfer you into an airline aisle chair to get you on and off the aircraft.

When changing planes, airport personnel will use another airport wheelchair to move you to the gate for boarding your next flight. It is generally not practical to have your own powered wheelchair brought up to the gate to change planes. Your chair would need to be reassembled and then disassembled, and the narrow stairways down to the aircraft from the jetway would make it very difficult to carry a powered wheelchair.

At some smaller airports, there may not be a jetway, but a stairway. Standard practice is to carry you down in the aisle chair. Some airports have a lift platform on a forklift. Newer technology lifts are being created to assist with getting on and off of smaller aircraft.

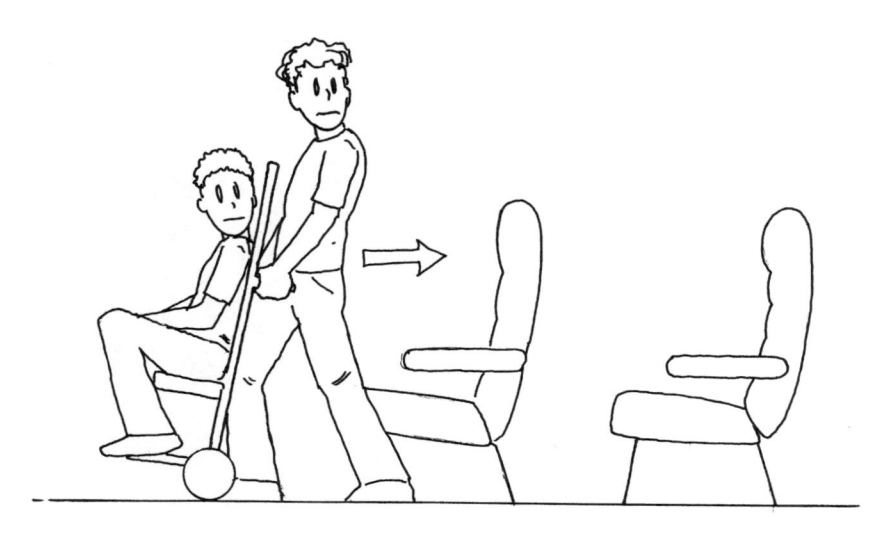

If needed, aisle chairs are narrow chairs designed for airline personnel to assist you on and off the aircraft.

Arriving at your destination

Once at your destination, make sure your wheelchair has been reassembled correctly and that it works before getting in it. If anything is broken or missing, speak immediately with a carrier representative for help. If you are worried about the handling of your mobility equipment, carry a copy of the Air Carriers Access Act regulations to help settle potential disputes, available through the Access Board in Washington D.C. If you travel with a service dog, pack a copy of your state regulations regarding service dog access, available from the office of your state's Attorney General.

CHAPTER 6

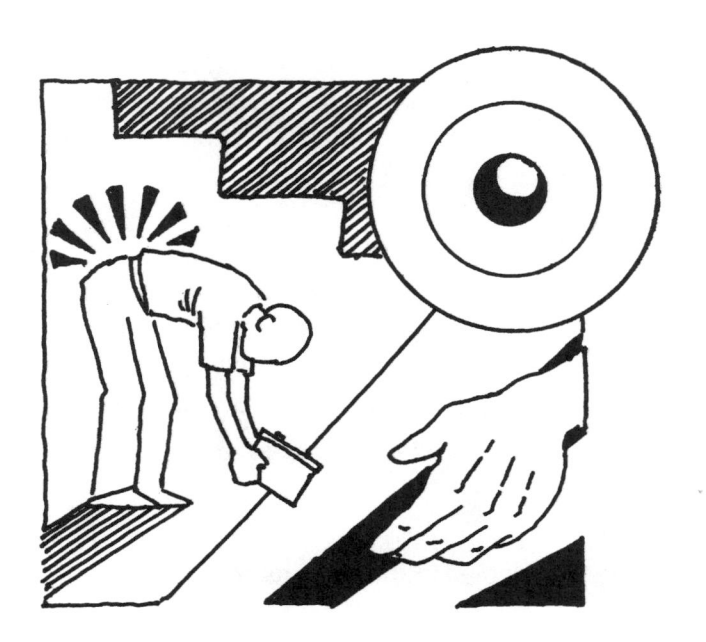

Body Mechanics

In this Chapter

6.1   Protecting Yourself　　　　　　　130

6.2   Setting Limits and Offering Help　　134

This chapter is meant as a guide for those who assist wheelchair riders. While lifting and pushing a wheelchair rider might not appear as risky as playing football or moving furniture, the types of injuries that may result can be identical. The wheelchair rider should also read this chapter to help protect spotters and assistants from injury. While reading this chapter, consider circumstances that will put you at risk for injury while helping a wheelchair user. Think of better ways to handle or avoid hazardous situations.

Before practicing the maneuvers in this chapter, read the warnings on page xi to learn about the risks involved. Remember that for some wheelchair riders, falling may result in severe injury or death, and that assisting a wheelchair rider could expose you to serious injury.

Chapter Six: Body Mechanics

Section 6.1

Protecting Yourself

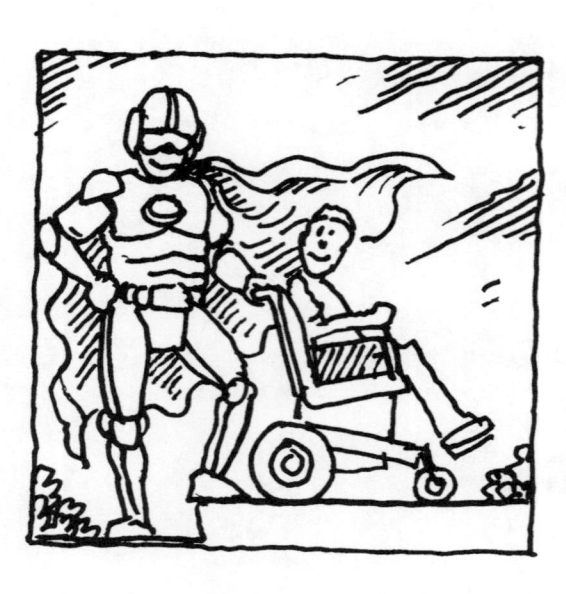

"Body mechanics" is a term used to describe the positioning and use of the body. Proper body mechanics when assisting a wheelchair rider can prevent injury. Common injuries include back strain and pulled muscles.

Body Position

Be aware of your body when you are assisting someone. If any part of your body hurts or feels awkward, you may not be positioned properly or you may have reached your physical limits. Stop and seek additional help.

Helping a wheelchair rider can require a lot of pushing, pulling and/or lifting. Always observe the following safe body mechanics principles to avoid straining your back.

- Bend your knees, not your waist.
- Keep your back upright and perpendicular to the floor as much as possible.
- Use your legs for strength rather than the weaker muscles of your back or stomach.
- Do not lock your knees.
- Never twist at the waist. Instead, keep your torso facing the same direction as your hips. Pivot your feet to change direction.
- Keep your back straight. Hunching over or rounding your shoulders can cause back strain.
- Keep breathing. Holding your breath stiffens your muscles, making them easier to injure.

Section 6.1: Protecting Yourself

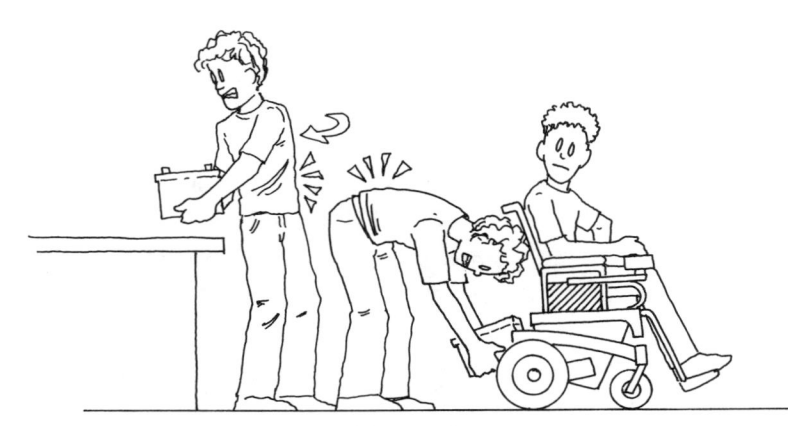

Twisting and bending at the waist can injure your back.

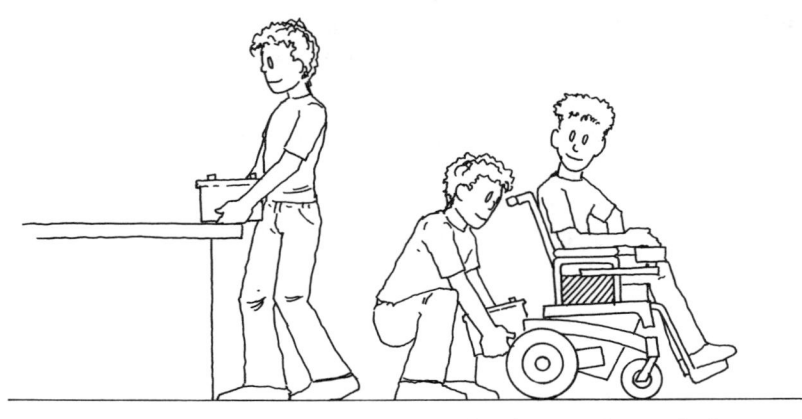

Bending at the knees and keeping your back straight can help you avoid injuring your back.

Using Safe Body Mechanics

Assisting up a curb going forward

- The wheelchair rider should position his or her chair to be facing the curb directly.

- As the primary assistant, you should be behind the wheelchair with your hands on the push handles, ready to provide additional forward power as the wheelchair rider drives forward up the curb.

- If the curb is too high for you to provide enough assistance, then identify a second assistant. When two assistants are available, the second assistant should stand to one side of the wheelchair and, while bending at the knees, grasp the frame of the wheelchair. Make sure the second assistant is not holding on to any removable parts. The second assistant should lift as the wheelchair rider drives forward up the curb.

With one assistant

- For this maneuver, it may be necessary to reposition or remove the anti-tippers so that they do not limit the amount the chair can tip.

- Position yourself behind the wheelchair with one foot in front of the other and grasp the push handles firmly.

- If necessary, push down on the push handles to help drive the casters up onto the curb.

- While the wheelchair rider drives forward, be ready to provide assistance by pushing the chair up the curb.

- Keep pushing on the wheelchair as needed until the rear wheels are up on the curb. Use your body weight to lean into the chair as you push forward.

- Use safe body mechanics when pushing by keeping your back straight and using your legs to power the push.

- When the maneuver is complete, reposition or reinstall the anti-tippers.

Chapter Six: Body Mechanics

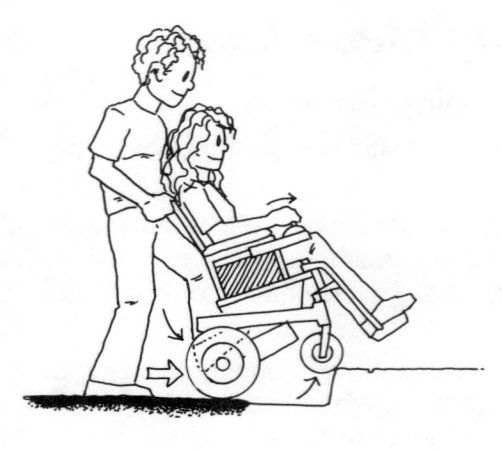

You can push down and back to help lift the casters onto the curb.

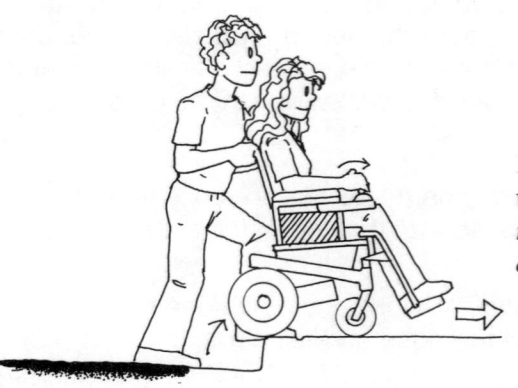

You can use your body weight to help push the rear wheels up onto the curb.

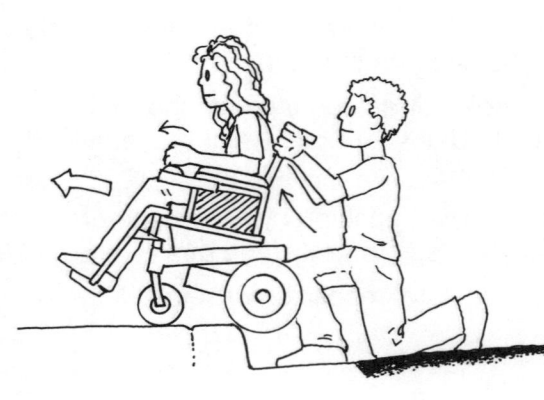

You can lower yourself to allow you to push the wheelchair up the curb with a straight back.

With two assistants

- For this maneuver, it may be necessary to reposition or remove the anti-tippers so that they do not limit the amount the chair can tip.
- Have the wheelchair rider drive forward to the curb until the foot supports or front casters are resting against it.
- Position yourself behind the wheelchair with one foot in front of the other and have the second assistant stand to the side of the wheelchair.
- The second assistant should grasp the frame of the wheelchair. Be sure that the assistant grasps a structural part of the wheelchair and not a removable part.
- On the wheelchair rider's count of three, use your body weight to lean into the chair as you push forward. The second assistant should lift and pull the front of the wheelchair while keeping a straight back. Have the wheelchair rider slowly drive the wheelchair forward.
- Be sure to use safe body mechanics by keeping your back straight and bending your knees to power the push and lift. You should feel your quadriceps muscles (located above your knee and up your thigh) working.
- When the maneuver is complete, reposition or reinstall the anti-tippers.

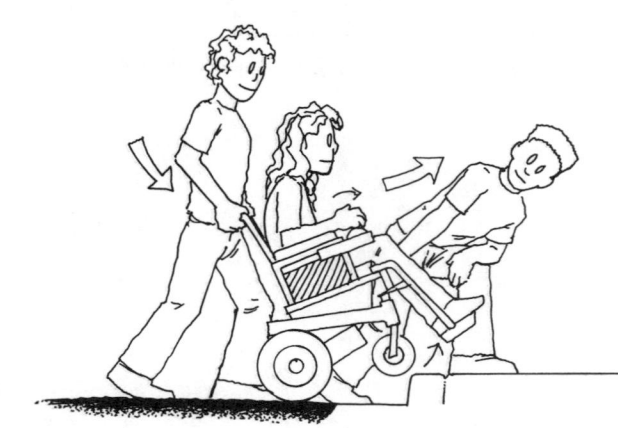

Using correct body mechanics makes the job easier and safer for you and the wheelchair rider.

Assisting down a curb going backward

- For this maneuver, it may be necessary to reposition or remove the anti-tippers so that they do not limit the amount the chair can tip.
- Have the wheelchair rider back up to the edge of the curb while you hold on to the push handles for safety.
- Stand behind the wheelchair, below the curb, with your hands on the push handles.
- Lean forward with your weight against the back of the wheelchair. Assist by controlling the descent as the wheelchair user slowly backs off the curb.
- Use your legs for strength and keep your back straight.
- When the maneuver is complete, reposition or reinstall the anti-tippers.

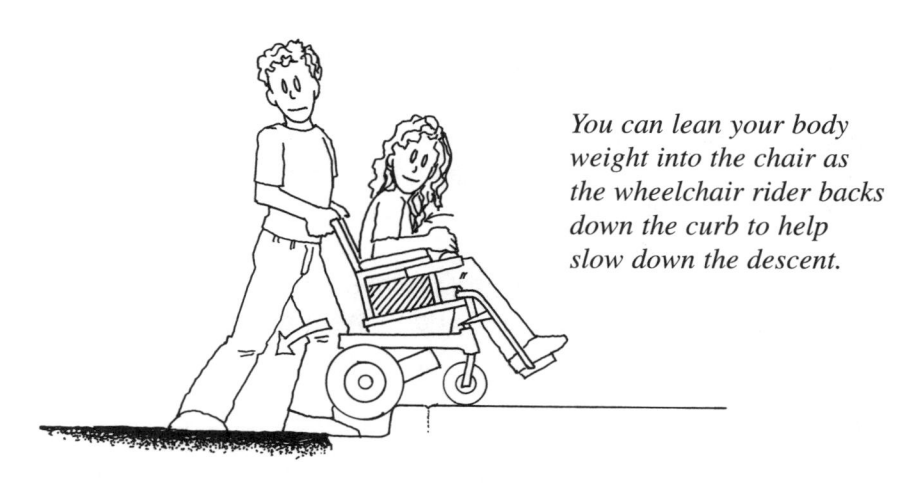

You can lean your body weight into the chair as the wheelchair rider backs down the curb to help slow down the descent.

Assisting through snow or sand

To help someone in a rear-wheel or mid-wheel drive chair, the most beneficial assistance is to reduce the weight on the front casters. To reduce the weight on the front casters, attach a belt or pull strap to the frame of the wheelchair near a front caster. You can use this belt or pull strap to assist the wheelchair through the soft surface. If a second assistant is available, have the second assistant push the wheelchair from behind while you lift up on the pull strap.

- Use a leather belt or some rope or webbing at least 2 to 3 feet long.
- Tie one end of the pull strap to a structural portion of the front of the wheelchair. Make sure it is not tied to a removable part.

With one assistant

- Stand slightly forward and to the side of the wheelchair.
- Reach back and grasp the pull strap, keeping your back straight and your elbows slightly bent.
- Lift up on the pull strap to unweight the front casters and pull the wheelchair forward while keeping your back straight and using your legs for power.
- Have the wheelchair user drive forward as you pull.

With two assistants

- Stand slightly forward and to the side of the wheelchair.
- Reach back and grasp the pull strap, keeping your back straight and your elbows slightly bent.
- Have the second assistant stand behind the wheelchair with one foot in front of the other and grasp the push handles firmly.
- Lift up on the pull strap to unweight the front casters and pull the wheelchair forward while keeping your back straight and using your legs for power. The second assistant should lean into the back of the wheelchair and push forward on the push handles, using his or her legs for power.
- Have the wheelchair user drive forward as you pull, and the second assistant pushes.
- Be sure you both keep your backs straight and use your legs for power.

Chapter Six: Body Mechanics

Section 6.2
Setting Limits and Offering Help

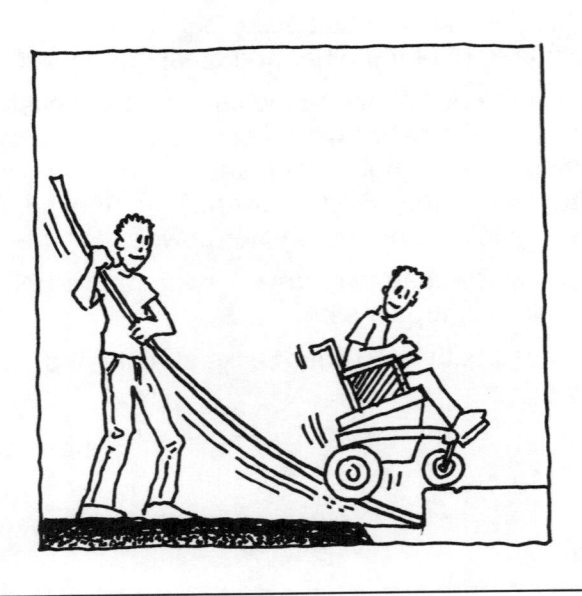

It can be hard to admit you have reached your limits. However, you should safeguard your own health and well-being. You need to know your limits and how to say "no" when you have reached them.

How to Say "No"

It is important to understand that you should not assist a wheelchair rider if it presents a physical hazard to your own health or you are not confident in the outcome. This could result in injury to the wheelchair rider and/or yourself. For example, pushing a wheelchair up a curb with an injured back could be painful and may cause further injury to your back. Do not be afraid to say "No." The following are several ways to decline to help:

- Politely decline by saying, "I don't feel comfortable or safe assisting you in that way." Explaining why you declined is often appreciated. However, if your reasons are personal, you have no obligation to explain yourself.
- Offer to find someone who can help. "I'm not able to assist you up this curb because I have a shoulder injury. Can I help you find someone else to assist?"
- Offer an alternative skill. "I'm not comfortable pulling your wheelchair backward up the curb because I don't think I can lift the weight of the wheelchair. Can we try lifting your casters up onto the curb and then I can push you up the curb?"
- Offer an alternative route. "I'm concerned about trying to assist you down this steep hill. The hill isn't so steep if we go to the next corner."

Offering Assistance

Sometimes watching a wheelchair rider do something is difficult because you can see that whatever the rider is doing is not easy. Remember that the person may not want assistance; it may be important for the person to accomplish the activity independently. It might be easier for the wheelchair rider to do the activity alone than to explain to others how they can help. The wheelchair rider might have had bad experiences or even injuries in the past when people tried to help. It may be difficult to watch, but you do not necessarily need to help the person.

Only assist a wheelchair rider when you are asked and/or have been given permission. If you think a wheelchair rider might need assistance, offer. The wheelchair rider may be in a position that looks precarious, but have the situation under control. Unexpected assistance might throw him or her off balance.

- Ask if the wheelchair user wants help. Avoid assertive statements such as, "Let me do this for you," which make it difficult for the wheelchair rider to decline your help.
- Try wording your offer more casually. "Could you use a hand?" or "Can I help you out?"

If your offer to assist has been accepted, let the wheelchair rider be in charge. Ask the wheelchair rider how you can help and follow the rider's instructions. Ask the wheelchair rider to talk you through the sequence before trying it, then work together to do it correctly.

- Do not push, lift or pull unless the wheelchair rider asks. Often you will be working together (e.g. to climb a curb, you may be pushing on the push handles as the wheelchair user drives forward).
- Speak up if you feel in danger of injuring yourself by following the rider's instructions.

Appendix A

The Americans with Disabilities Act of 1990

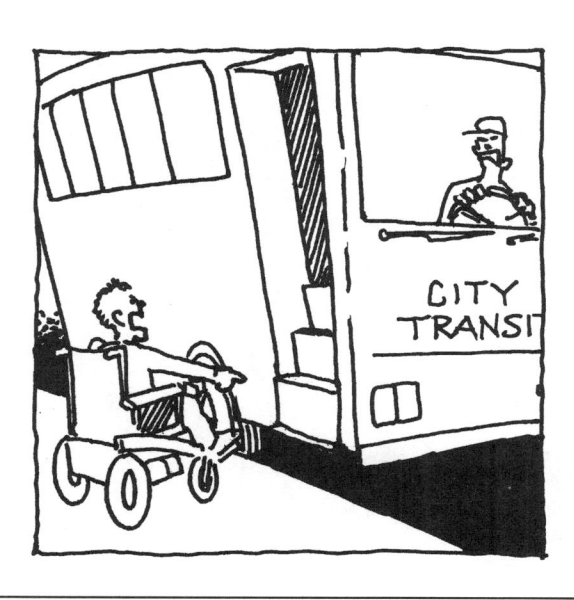

The Americans with Disabilities Act (ADA) was adopted as law in 1990 to ensure that equal access is provided to all individuals without regard to needs related to disability. This comprehensive law focuses on a number of areas, including accessibility to and within public buildings and services.

If you encounter problems with the accessibility of a building, you should first speak with the building owner or manager and explain your problem. They may have been unaware of any accessibility difficulties, and could make immediate changes for you. If the building manager or owner is unwilling to help, the next step is to get other people in the building to talk to the management. Local advocacy groups, such as Centers for Independent Living, may offer intermediary services or provide alternative resources for addressing problems. If you cannot achieve a resolution of the problem using these methods, you can file a complaint with the Department of Justice. For information about filing a complaint, call the ADA information line at 800-514-0301.

A problem might be as simple as a plant that was placed in front of the elevator buttons or within the clear passage of a hallway. It may be as complex as a multi-level building not serviced by an elevator or doorways that are too narrow for you to pass through.

U.S. Department of Justice

The U.S. Department of Justice provides general information about the Americans with Disabilities Act (ADA), answers to specific technical questions, ADA materials, and information about filing a complaint.

websites	www.usdoj.gov/disabilities.htm
	www.usdoj.gov/crt/ada/adahom1.htm
ADA Information Line	Voice 800-514-0301
	TTY 800-514-0383

The Access Board

The U.S. Architectural and Transportation Barriers Compliance Board (The Access Board) provides technical assistance on the ADA Accessibility Guidelines.

website	www.access-board.gov
Voice	800-872-2253
TTY	800-993-2822

U.S. Department of Transportation

The ADA also addresses accessibility to transportation services. The U.S. Department of Transportation oversees this aspect of the ADA.

website   www.dot.gov/accessibility

Office of the Secretary
Office of Civil Rights   Voice   202-366-4648
   TTY   202-366-5273

Federal Transit Administration
Office of Civil Rights   Voice   888-446-4511
   E-mail   ada.assistance@fta.dot.gov

Appendix B

Specialty Powered Wheelchairs and Accessories

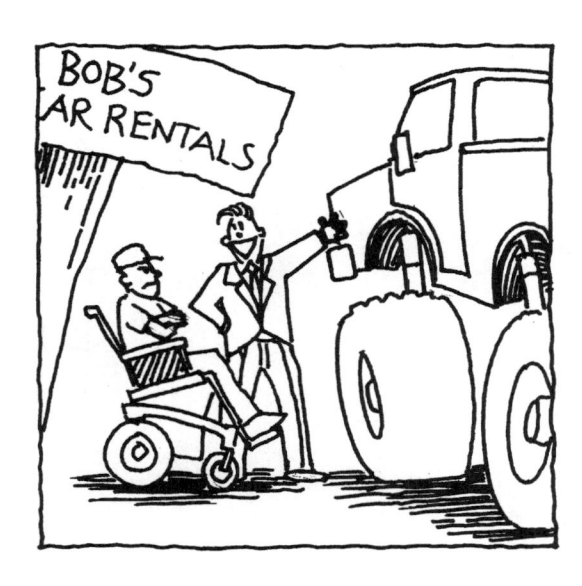

The availability of specialty wheelchairs and accessories has expanded tremendously. Specialty wheelchairs usually allow you to do specific things really well, like maneuver indoors in tight spaces. However, the same specialty wheelchair would usually not work as well outdoors.

You could never need or use all the accessories available on the market – if you did, your chair would be bristling with enough gadgets and gizmos to rival a one-man novelty band. The accessories you choose to use will reflect your function and the things you want to do. An accessory you use all the time might be merely a hindrance to someone else. You will grow out of some accessories you found indispensable when you first started using a wheelchair. You may find other accessories beneficial as you gain experience.

Below is a list of different specialty wheelchairs and accessories, including a description, other common terms for each accessory, and the positives and negatives of some of them.

Some of the specialty wheelchairs are not available in some countries or were not on the market yet at the time this was written. Hopefully, they will give you an idea of what is possible.

WARNING!

Many powered wheelchair accessories are designed to increase the visibility of your chair in outdoor environments. Reflectors, lighting, flags, mirrors and horns will not guarantee your safety if you choose to operate your powered wheelchair in an environment shared by motor vehicles. A powered wheelchair is no match against a car, van or truck in a collision. In a powered wheelchair, you are traveling at a fairly slow speed and do not have the ability to drive up a curb or jump out of the chair to get off of the roadway. Always be aware that you are taking an extreme risk if you choose to operate your wheelchair in a vehicular environment. Many manual and powered wheelchair users have been killed while operating their chairs in the roadway.

Appendix B: Specialty Powered Wheelchairs and Accessories

add-on power system – designed to convert a manual wheelchair into a powered wheelchair. Some add-on power systems attach to the front of the wheelchair and have a single drive wheel just behind the foot supports. Another type connects onto the back of the wheelchair and has drive motors that drive the rear wheels by friction.

- Plus: easier to disassemble for travel than standard powered wheelchair motors; can provide power assistance driving up a hill or over long distances while still permitting the chair to be used in manual mode
- Minus: added weight significantly decreases the maneuverability of the manual wheelchair in manual mode

airless tire insert, flat-free insert – designed to fit inside the tire to eliminate the need for air-filled tubes; usually made of foam.

- Plus: eliminates the risk of sustaining a flat tire
- Minus: usually result in a rougher ride than air-filled tires; more difficult and expensive to change when tire wears out

anti-tippers – small wheels attached to the back of many rear-wheel drive wheelchairs, designed to prevent you from tipping over backward. Anti-tippers are often included with your wheelchair equipment.

- Plus: allows you to climb steep hills with a reduced risk of completely tipping over backwards
- Minus: limits the ability to cross and climb obstacles and curbs; they do not always prevent a powered chair from tipping over

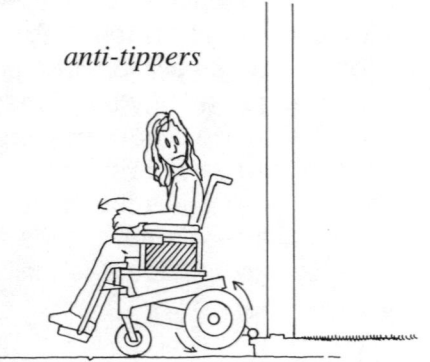

anti-tippers

arm support panel – plastic or metal guard that attaches to the arm support, between the wheel and the rider.

- Plus: keeps tire dirt on the outside of arm support and away from your clothes
- Minus: may reduce the effective width of your wheelchair seat; be sure to check the pressure on both sides of your hip bones

backpack – bag designed to be worn on the back that can also be attached to the back of a wheelchair by hooking the straps over the push handles or frame. Backpacks specifically designed for wheelchairs are also available.

- Plus: can carry an assortment of supplies
- Minus: additional weight on the back of the chair can increase the likelihood of tipping over backward (if you plan to use a backpack often, practice skills with it on your chair)

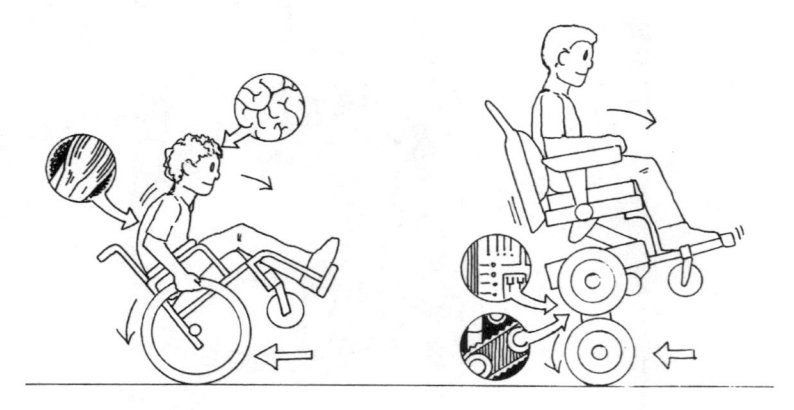

balancing wheelchair – powered wheelchair with gyros that maintain the balance of the wheelchair. This technology allows the user to balance and feel like they are standing up.

balancing wheelchair

beach wheelchair (powered)
– wheelchair designed to negotiate sand and soft surfaces; has wider tires with a larger tread pattern and a longer wheelbase to provide added stability. Since many recreation areas do not allow motorized vehicles, three- and four-wheelers have been converted into powered beach wheelchairs without the noise and pollution of the motorized ATV.

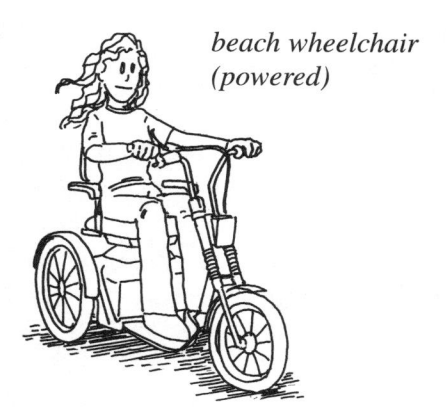

beach wheelchair (powered)

bicycle light – light designed to clip onto bicycles; can increase your visibility to motorists, cyclists and others. A white halogen lamp can act as a headlight. Blinking red lights can be clipped to the rear of your wheelchair to improve your visibility from the rear.

- Plus: helps you view upcoming terrain, increases your visibility to motorists, cyclists and others when traveling in the street at night; removable
- Minus: may not be as easy to mount on a wheelchair as it is to mount to a bike; adding bicycle lights to the chair does not guarantee safety in the street environment – a powered wheelchair is no match against a motor vehicle

bike trailer – wheeled cart that can be attached to the back of the wheelchair for added storage.

- Plus: adds storage space if you need to transport a lot of things
- Minus: limits maneuverability, uses more energy to drive the wheelchair

cellular phone – portable, wireless telephone.

- Plus: can be used to contact help in an emergency
- Minus: must keep batteries charged; could possibly cause electromagnetic interference – see Section 4.3

chest strap – strap attached to the back of the wheelchair that crosses under your arms and over your chest. It can help prevent you from falling forward. Always use a lap belt if you are using a chest strap.

- Plus: can prevent injury that might occur when falling forward out of wheelchair during sudden stops; provides additional trunk stability
- Minus: locks you into your wheelchair; can restrict mobility of trunk and/or buttocks; use of a chest support without a lap belt could result in strangulation if the user slides down in the wheelchair; lap belt should be mounted at a 60 to 90 degree angle to the seat in order to prevent user from sliding down in the chair

clothing guard, mud guard – plastic or nylon guard that stays between your wheel and clothes to keep you clean.

- Plus: keeps clothing from getting soiled by dirt kicked up from tires
- Minus: some people find clothing guards unsightly; may narrow the width of the seat

duct tape – wide plastic tape embedded with fiber webbing for strength.

- Plus: very strong and sticky; can be used for temporary repairs while on the road
- Minus: should not be used in place of proper wheelchair parts (e.g. not equivalent to a bolt); may leave a sticky residue after removal

electrical tape – thin, stretchy plastic tape that is used to bind electrical wires; available in many colors.

Appendix B: Specialty Powered Wheelchairs and Accessories

Plus: can be used for temporary on-the-road repairs until you can get the problem fixed properly

Minus: not as sticky or strong as duct tape

elevating seat system – powered wheelchair seat that rises up and down; many powered chairs are available with elevating seats. The maximum speed of the chair usually reduces when the seat is elevated.

flag – tall, flexible rod with a triangular flag (usually vinyl or plastic); usually comes in a fluorescent color; can be mounted to the back of your wheelchair to improve your visibility.

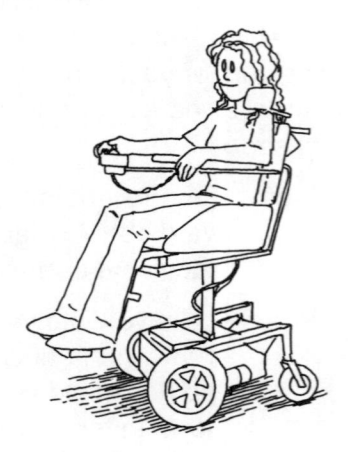

Plus: helps make you more visible to motorists

elevating seat system

Minus: many dislike the way the flag looks; can get caught on low hanging obstacles; adding a flag to the chair does not guarantee safety in the street environment – the powered wheelchair is no match against a motor vehicle

flashlight – useful when traveling along dark streets and to improve your visibility to others. For easy access, use a Velcro™ strap to attach it to the frame of your wheelchair. Better yet, you can attach a bicycle light to your wheelchair to see the path in front of your chair. A head lamp allows you to see in front of you.

Plus: can be used to look for lost objects and to help perform emergency repairs

Minus: people with limited hand function may have difficulty operating; adding a flashlight to the chair does not guarantee safety in the street environment – a powered wheelchair is no match against a motor vehicle

foot straps – straps that attach to the foot supports and loop over the top of each foot to keep them from sliding forward off the foot supports.

Plus: prevent feet from falling forward off foot supports; limit the chance of injury or accident caused by your feet hitting the ground in front of the foot supports; help prevent legs from falling into your face in a backward fall

Minus: need to be released for transfers

golf cart – single-person golf carts can be used as a personal mobility device for softer surfaces.

Plus: good for traveling on softer surfaces

Minus: not useful for indoor mobility

golf cart

hand wipes, wet naps, baby wipes – wet cloths used for cleaning hands and face; available in plastic dispensers or individual packets.

Plus: can clean your hands when a sink is not nearby or accessible

head support – postural support device that mounts to the back of the wheelchair and is used to support the head.

Plus: reduces chance of whiplash if head is snapped back when riding in a vehicle

Minus: may limit sight when looking behind; may not help prevent whiplash in an accident; may make it difficult to enter or exit a van without raised doors

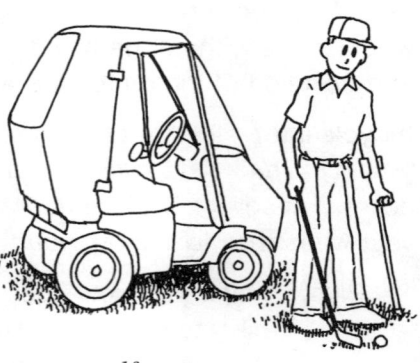

indoor-only wheelchair – a powered wheelchair specially designed for maneuvering indoors in tight spaces but not for outdoor travel.

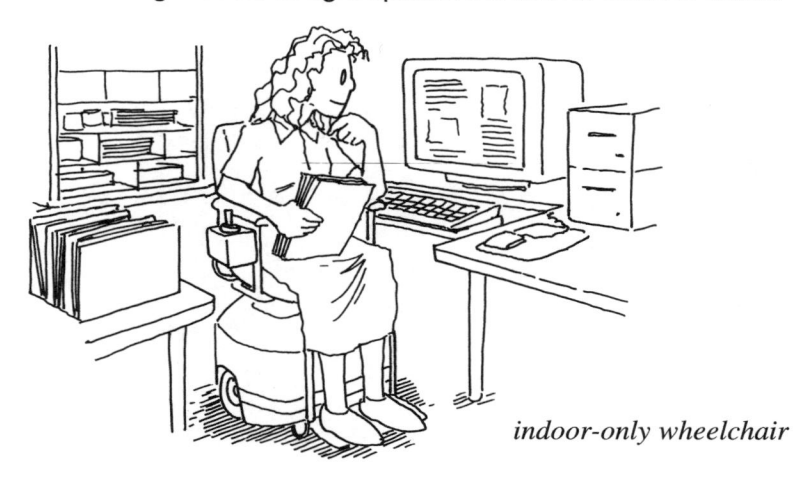

indoor-only wheelchair

key clasp – small clasp with key rings attached that can hook keys to the frame of the wheelchair.

    Plus: easy access to keys; keeps keys visible to limit theft

    Minus: clasp may be hard to open for persons with limited hand function

lap belt – belt worn across the lap to prevent forward falls out of the wheelchair. A lap belt should always be used when using a chest support to prevent you from sliding down in your wheelchair. Lap belts come in many different styles.

    Plus: can prevent injury that might occur when falling forward out of the wheelchair due to a sudden stop; provides stability

> **WARNING!**
> Lap belts are not designed nor intended to be used as a restraint (seat belt) in a motor vehicle.

    Minus: an improperly mounted lap belt can create a strangulation hazard if the user slides under the belt; lap belts should be mounted such that when in use they create a 60 to 90 degree angle to the seat

lap tray – flat removable surface (usually plastic) that mounts to the wheelchair frame and extends over your lap. It can be used as a surface for eating, playing games, reading, writing, etc.

    Plus: can provide a good substitute for a table when tables and counters are too low

    Minus: adds weight; may feel and look awkward; limits the ability to access other areas

leg strap – strap that positions the legs within the wheelchair frame. There is usually one strap behind the legs; less common is a second strap in front of the legs.

    Plus: prevents feet from falling off foot supports, limiting chance of injury caused by the feet getting stuck behind the foot supports; useful on rough terrain

    Minus: may interfere with swing-away foot supports

lowering seat – seat that lowers user to the floor. Some powered wheelchairs are designed to allow the user to get down to the floor to get in and out of the wheelchair or to interact with others.

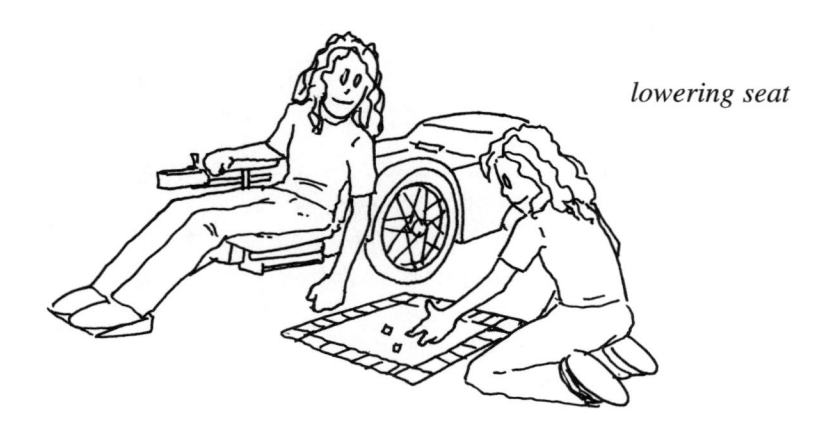

lowering seat

Appendix B: Specialty Powered Wheelchairs and Accessories

luggage carriers – small lever arms that attach to the leg supports to create a ledge when folded down. When folded down, they can hold a briefcase or travel bag at your feet, where you can access it easily. They fold up and out of the way when not in use.

- Plus: keeps items conveniently located; fold up when not in use
- Minus: a heavy bag could tip the wheelchair forward; a heavy load on the front of the chair could lower the foot supports on the chair and cause them to catch on the ground, bringing the chair to an abrupt stop and possibly throwing you forward out of the chair

mirror – mirror mounted onto the frame of your wheelchair. A mirror can be used like a rearview mirror on a car.

- Plus: helps you see what's behind you
- Minus: will not help you see what is in your blind spot (the area just to the side and behind you that is not reflected in the mirror); adding a mirror to the chair does not guarantee safety in the street environment – a powered wheelchair is no match against a motor vehicle

noisemaker – horn or bell attached to your wheelchair. A noisemaker can be purchased at bicycle shops and can be used to signal motorists, pedestrians, and bicyclists.

- Plus: notifies other motorists, pedestrians, and bicyclists of your presence to reduce the possibility of a collision
- Minus: some do not like the way horns look or sound; may be difficult to reach and activate; adding a noisemaker to the chair does not guarantee safety in the street environment – a powered wheelchair is no match against a motor vehicle

off-road wheelchair – powered wheelchair with large, knobbed tires, similar to those found on mountain bikes, featuring a longer wheelbase for improved stability. Off-road wheelchairs are designed to negotiate rough, unpaved surfaces. The length of some off-road wheelchairs is adjustable to improve indoor mobility.

off-road wheelchair

- Plus: permits you to access more types of surfaces
- Minus: often heavier and requires more battery power than a standard powered wheelchair

power-assist wheelchair – powered wheelchair that is set up to be controlled by the attendant or caregiver.

power-assist wheelchair

pump – device used to inflate tires with air.

- Plus: handy in the event of an emergency

push handles – handles attached to the top of the seat back that enable an assistant to push or tilt the wheelchair.

- Plus: helpful if assistance is required frequently; can be used as an elbow hook for stability or to help right yourself after leaning forward to perform a weight shift; will usually hit the ground first if you tip over backward, which could help protect your head

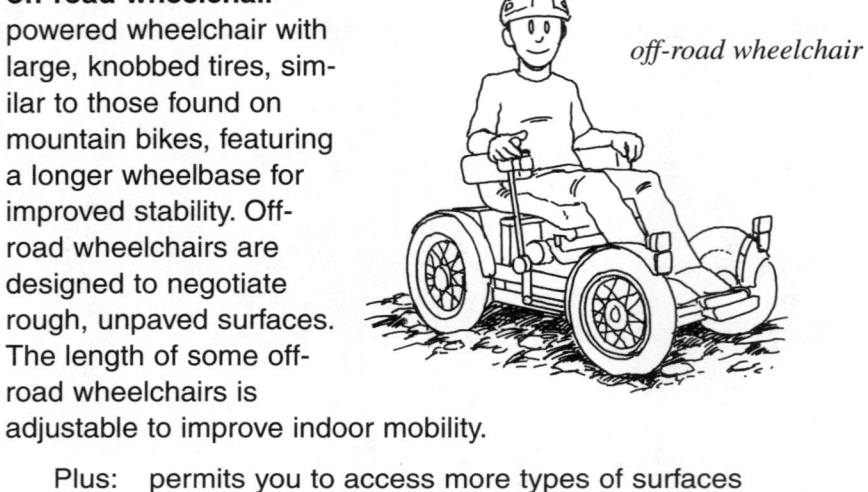

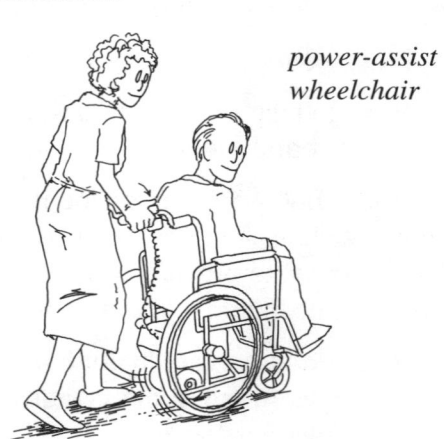

144

recliner, reclining back support – back support with an adjustable angle that allows the seat-to-back angle to be increased; may come with or without elevating leg supports.

recliner, reclining back support

- Plus: can be used to stretch, to perform a weight shift, or for postural stability; may help with bed to wheelchair transfers (recline back support and roll or slide from bed onto your wheelchair); elevating leg supports can help to increase blood circulation in the legs

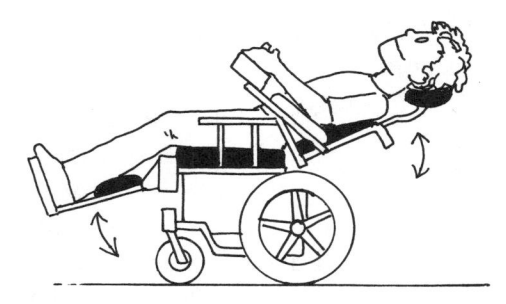

- Minus: chairs with recliners often have long wheelbases for stability, which increases the turning space required and decreases the maneuverability of the wheelchair; are a little heavier than standard powered wheelchairs

recreational accessories – any accessory added to a wheelchair to enhance recreational activity. Powered wheelchairs can be modified for various types of recreational activities. To play powered wheelchair soccer, low friction front and side bumpers are attached to the frame of the wheelchair. Other kinds of modifications are done for other sports.

recreational accessories

reflector – plastic disk or rectangle that reflects light aimed at it. Reflectors can be attached to the spokes, frame, or back of a wheelchair to improve your visibility to motorists. Brightly colored plastic or vinyl tape that reflects light can also be attached to your wheelchair and/or clothing.

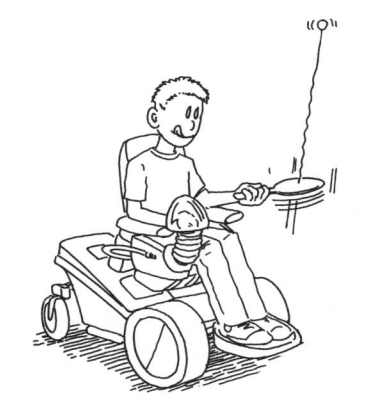

- Plus: makes you more visible to motorists and cyclists with lights

- Minus: depending on how it is attached, it may appear unsightly to some wheelchair users; reflectorizing the chair does not guarantee safety in the street environment – a powered wheelchair is no match against a motor vehicle

seat cushion – cushioning for a wheelchair seat. Seat cushions come in a variety of styles and materials, including plastic, foam, gel, air, and water. Custom cushions can be made to fit your body. Select the appropriate cushion type after consulting with a rehabilitation or seating therapist.

- Plus: a proper seat cushion can improve posture and comfort and may lessen the potential of developing of pressure ulcers

- Minus: a seat cushion not suited to your needs may adversely affect your posture and stability and cause pressure ulcers

seat pouch – cloth pouch specifically designed to be attached under wheelchair seats. A fanny pack (nylon or cloth pouches worn around the waist) can be modified to serve as a seat pouch.

- Plus: provides additional storage space; under-seat position may provide better security than a backpack

- Minus: people with little or no upper body strength may have difficulty reaching a seat pouch

shoulder harness – strap that fits over your shoulders and hooks around the back of a wheelchair to help keep you upright and bolster your forward stability.

- Plus: can prevent injury that might occur when falling forward out of your wheelchair

Minus: may limit reach; use of a shoulder harness without a lap belt or with an improperly mounted one, could result in strangulation if the user slides down in the wheelchair

stair climbing wheelchair – wheelchair or wheelchair carrier that allows a wheelchair user to go up and down stairs. Some models allow independent use, while others require the assistance of an attendant. Some use tracks and others use two or three-wheel clusters. Most of these chairs are only marketed in Europe.

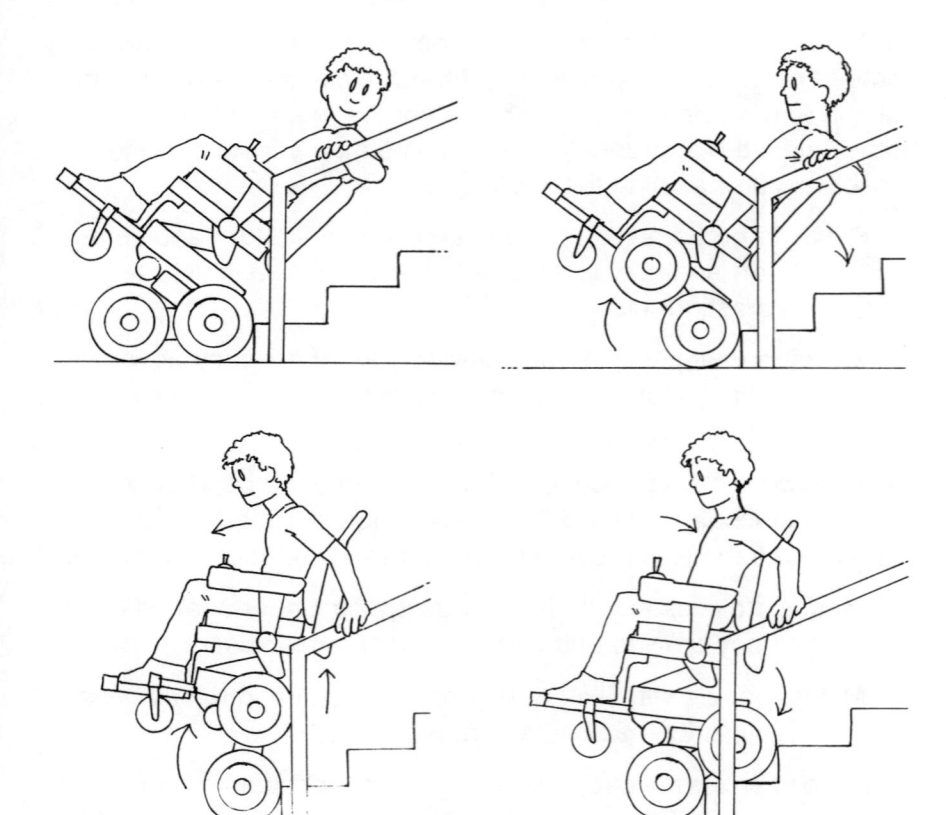

stair climbing wheelchair

standing wheelchair – wheelchair that stands the user in an upright position.

Plus: helps wheelchair users stand to perform functional tasks; allows you to stretch your muscles; allows your bladder to drain better; other benefits of standing are being researched

standing wheelchair

Swiss army knife (or other multi-purpose tool) – functions as an all-in-one tool kit. Depending on the model, it can also include a screw driver, scissors, knife blades, files, pliers and tweezers.

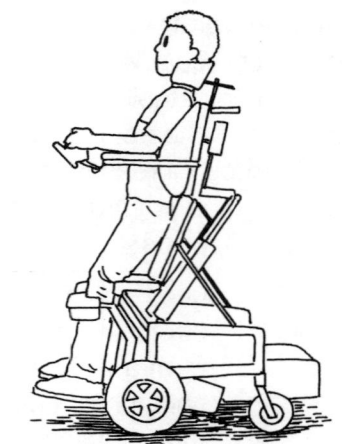

Plus: handy while out and about, saves time spent looking for tools

Minus: requires good hand function to operate; is not allowed through airport security

terrain-following wheelchair – wheelchair that has the ability to sense the slope it is on and reposition the seating to keep the user upright.

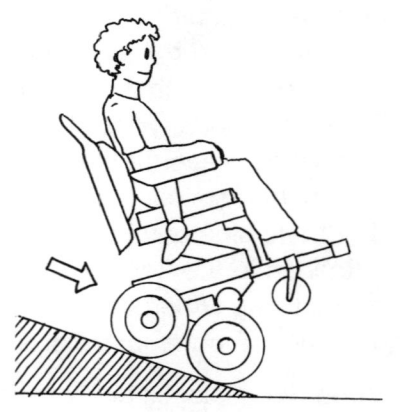

terrain-following wheelchair

tilt-in-space – seating system that allows you to change the orientation of the seat on the frame by adjusting the angle of the back support and the seat together as one unit.

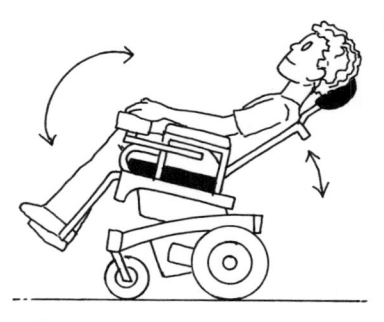

tilt-in-space

- Plus: can be used to perform a weight shift; can provide additional postural stability; can increase sitting time

- Minus: chairs with tilt-in-space may have longer wheelbases for stability; a longer wheelbase increases the turning space required and decreases the maneuverability of the wheelchair

trunk supports – postural support devices that can be added to a wheelchair back to improve the sitting position of the user. May include lateral or side-to-side supports.

- Plus: provides stability

- Minus: may restrict mobility of trunk; may interfere with transfers

Appendix C

References and Resources

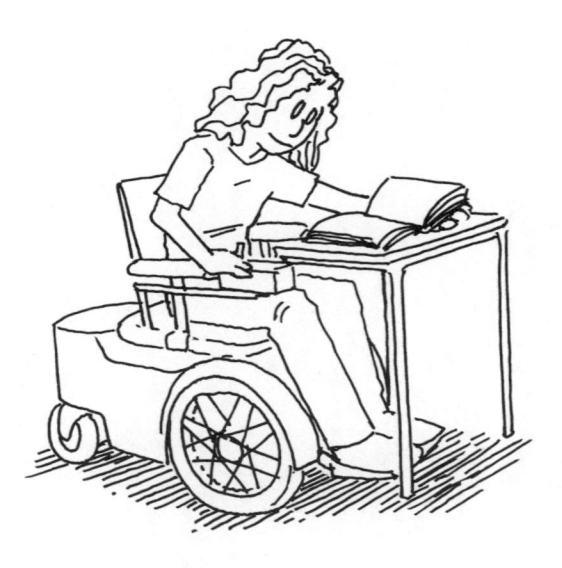

If you are interested in obtaining additional information about wheelchairs and mobility skills, there are a number of resources you can tap with a visit, a phone call, a letter or a modem.

Centers for Independent Living (CIL)

Most communities have a Center for Independent Living (also called Independent Living Centers or ILCs). These centers are run by and for people with disabilities. Their mission is to help people with disabilities live more independently and become productive, fully participating members of society.

Rehabilitation Centers

The rehabilitation center in your area may have facilities you can use to try out equipment and see which devices might benefit you. They may recommend an evaluation by an occupational or physical therapist, or a RESNA certified assistive technology practitioner. These professionals can often provide you with insight into your abilities and potential needs, and may be able to direct you toward other helpful accessories. Your rehabilitation center may also refer you to other centers that can better meet your specific needs.

Medical Equipment Suppliers

Medical Equipment Suppliers represent equipment manufacturers and should be able to help you make equipment choices compatible with your lifestyle. Remember that these companies are in the business of selling equipment, so you need to be an educated consumer and look further than the salesperson. The National Registry of Rehabilitation Technology Suppliers has a registry of equipment suppliers.

When buying equipment, consider the resources and reliability of the supplier. Ask them about their repair policies. For instance, will they loan you equipment when yours is being repaired? Are they helpful on the telephone? Do they seem willing to spend time telling you about the pros and cons of the variety of equipment? Will they help you adjust and re-adjust your equipment? The supplier should be willing to give you the names of a few of their

Appendix C: References and Resources

customers. Contact these people to determine how they feel about the supplier's services.

Equipment Manufacturers

Most wheelchair and related equipment manufacturers have toll-free numbers and are available for assistance. They will often refer you to a local supplier or others in your area who are familiar with their products. Some manufacturers have technical assistance departments that may be able to help you with specific questions about modifications, adjustments or repairs. Some manufacturers publish documents in addition to their wheelchair owner's manuals. You can talk with your local supplier about getting documents from any of the manufacturers.

Other Users

Find people in your community who have similar interests and needs. Other people often have recommendations for equipment and you can combine their information with the recommendations you get from rehab professionals and equipment suppliers. By learning as much as you can, you will be able to make informed decisions about your equipment.

Professional Organizations

Some professional organizations may be able to provide you with information directly or refer you to members in your area who may be familiar with similar circumstances to yours.

APTA
American Physical Therapy Association
1111 N. Fairfax St. (800) 999-2782
Alexandria, VA 22314 www.apta.org

AOTA
American Occupational Therapy Association
4720 Montgomery Lane (800) 729-2682
PO Box 31220 www.aota.org
Bethesda, MD 20824-1220 info@aota.org

NRRTS
National Registry of Rehabilitation Technology Suppliers
P.O. Box 4033 (512) 267-6832
Lago Vista, TX 78645-4033 www.nrrts.org
 nrrts@ctsinet.com

Paralyzed Veterans of America
Spinal Cord Injury Education and Training Foundation
801 18th Street NW (800) 424-8200
Washington, DC 20006 www.pva.org
 info@pva.org

RESNA
Rehabilitation Engineering and Assistive Technology Society of North America
1700 N. Moore St., Suite 1540 (703) 524-6686
Arlington, VA 22209-1903 www.resna.org
 info@resna.org

Appendix C: References and Resources

Publications

A Guide to Wheelchair Selection: How to Use the ANSI/RESNA Wheelchair Standards to Buy a Wheelchair
Written by Peter Axelson, Jean Minkel and Denise Chesney
Paralyzed Veterans of America, Washington, DC
PVA Publications Distribution Center   (888) 860-7244
info@pva.org

Active Living Magazine
P.O. Box 2659
Niagara Falls, NY 14302-9945
www.cripworld.com/themall/activeliving/shtml

Enable Magazine
Magazine of the American Association of People
with Disabilities (AAPD)   (800) 840-8844
1819 H Street NW,
Suite 300   www.dnaco.net/~elainc/enable.html
Washington, DC 20006   readenable@aol.com

New Mobility
No Limits, Inc.
P.O. Box 220   (888) 850-0344
Horsham, PA 19044   www.newmobility.com

Paraplegia News
PVA Publications   (606) 224-0500
2111 East Highland Avenue, Suite 180   www.pn-magazine.com
Phoenix, AZ 85016-4702   pvapub@aol.com

Sports 'n Spokes
PVA Publications   (602) 224-0500
2111 East Highland Avenue, Suite 180   www.sns-magazine.com
Phoenix, AZ 85016-4702   pvapub@aol.com
Sports 'n Spokes publishes articles comparing available wheelchair models.

Websites

There are numerous websites with information about wheelchairs and for wheelchair users. Here are a few of them.

ABLEDATA
www.abledata.com
A searchable database of rehabilitation products.

Beneficial Designs, Inc.
www.beneficialdesigns.com
A rehabilitation engineering design firm specializing in recreational technologies, innovative wheeled mobility and seating, and access to outdoor recreation environments.

SpinLife
www.SpinLife.com
A site featuring wheelchairs, scooters and accessories.

WheelchairJunkie
www.WheelchairJunkie.com
A site for wheelchair users by wheelchair users.

WheelchairNet
www.WheelchairNet.org
A virtual community that provides information, support and a forum for wheelchair users.